# *Preface*

We first published this book in 1983, Our goal was to include tennis in the "fitness revolution" that was sweeping the country at that time. The most popular aspect of this new attitude was cardiovascular fitness. Hence the question for tennis players was, "Can playing tennis raise my heart rate?"

Shortly after publication of *Aerobic Tennis,* Dr. Bob Arnett of NBC invited me to New York City during the U.S. Open to demonstrate Aerobic Tennis. He wanted to know if his heart rate could be substantially raised by playing tennis. Dr. Bob and I did an experiment on the stadium court at the West Side Tennis Court. The idea was to compare typical aerobic exercise routines with using tennis for an aerobic workout.

I asked Bob to raise his heart rate on his own by running the stairs of the stadium and sprinting along the court. He ran for 3 or 4 minutes and we measured his heart rate. He rested to get his heart rate back to normal. Then we went out on the court with a basket of balls. I had him play points with no rest in between for 3 or 4 minutes. I pushed him: making him run, jump, and stretch for balls–simulating a vigorous and energetic game of tennis. Then we measured his heart rate, and voila! His rate was substantially higher than when he ran the stadium stairs. Plus he had more fun!

That afternoon of tennis was noted by the United States Tennis Association: they endorsed a "Cardio Tennis" program among their membership and successfully sponsored "Cardio Tennis" classes at hundreds of clubs across the United States–using tennis to improve aerobic fitness.

There's more. Tennis can do more than improve cardiovascular fitness. Tennis is the perfect form of interval training, with ebbs and flows of activity and rest. In this it's similar to the *fartlek* method of training developed by Swedish distance runners, which utilizes bursts of vigorous activity followed by rest.

Tennis offers other fitness benefits. Strength is developed when you try to increase racquet head speed on serves and ground strokes. Your balance is tested when you hit a ball, and then must return quickly to retrieve another one. Only the most agile of athletes is able to respond to hitting a ball at different heights and speeds from unpredictable and challenging positions.

We were ahead of our time in the '80s. Now, some 28 years later, "Cardio Tennis" is a well-known concept, and it utilizes the exact same principles that are in this book.

We're happy to present this concept again and hope that *Aerobic Tennis* will show you how to maximize physical fitness while engaging in the sport you love. This wholesome game challenges you athletically, so turn the athlete inside you loose! You can become a pitcher, a shortstop, a goalie, and a sprinter. Let your imagination run wild!

# *Introduction*

*In this age of fitness consciousness,* people are no longer trying to work as *little* as possible and expend the *least* amount of physical energy. Instead, they are looking for ways to tax themselves physically, for interesting ways to exercise, for new challenges. They know that the effort of an hour's aerobic exercise will make the next 12 hours so much more enjoyable because they'll be energized and feel more alive.

Yet tennis players with fitness goals often seem to turn to other activities—to running, bicycling, swimming, aerobic dancing—to get a stimulating workout. Many even give up tennis in frustration: "I get a better sweat playing racquetball," or "I just don't get a good workout," or "It's not good aerobic exercise like running."

Why is this? Perhaps because tennis has traditionally been thought of as a country club sport where sweat was inappropriate and the idea was to make it look easy. Players have been so concerned with a "look," with style, technique, or winning that they've overlooked the physical aspects of the game and the chance to get a good workout. What a mistake!

Tennis—with a new approach—can give you a superb aerobic workout, and improve your overall fitness, your strength and your agility. Playing tennis gives you the chance to:

- Run, leap, lunge and stretch.

- Work your major body muscles.

- Get your heart pumping strongly and improve your cardio-vascular fitness.

At the same time, tennis has these advantages over "just plain exercise"; it gives you:

- The excitement of the bouncing ball to keep you moving.

- The mental stimulation of strategy and tactics.

- The camaraderie and competition of a friend or opponent.

*Aerobic Tennis* is where the game of tennis finally catches up with the fitness revolution. It's a brand new look at a grand old game. Instead of tying yourself in knots over the details of technique, trying to look like someone else, or at the other extreme "working" to relax, you're going to go out on the court and involve your whole body in everything you do. At the same time, you are going to learn how to orient your off-court sports and activities to make you a more fit athlete and a better tennis player.

I developed the *Aerobic Tennis* method over 30 years of watching, teaching and coaching players of all ages and levels of skill. I began to notice that with every player who had a consistently good shot—whether at Wimbledon or down at the local Berkeley courts—there were some common elements:

- The whole body was behind the shot: the more body, the better the shot.

- The player was getting *away* from the ball so he or she could move *into* the ball with weight and power.

- The player wasn't concerned with technicalities and wasn't worried about overworked slogans like "Get your racket back," or "Get sideways to the net," or "Scratch your back."

- The racket appeared to be an extension of the body.

- The entire stroke was a continuous rhythmic expression.

These players all seemed to enjoy the running, the jumping, the reaching and the exertion of the game. They looked forward to hitting the ball. They didn't dread the ball coming over the net, they *wanted* it to come back so they could hit it again.

Comparing my students to these players, I began to realize that I was over-teaching and over-coaching. I was breaking the strokes down into too many elements. It was like teaching by the numbers. It was producing a very mechanical result, unlike the spontaneous, flowing strokes of good players.

I then started looking for a teaching technique that would allow the player to put as much of himself or herself into the shot as possible. I began experimenting with the club players in Vail, Colorado one summer and with my team at the University of California at Berkeley.

Laurie was a typical player in Vail who tried to muscle the ball with her arm; the harder she tried the worse she became. Marty Davis, three-time All-American at Cal had the same problem, but on a different level. With both players there was a need to make the arm part of a complete body action, rather than an isolated movement. The trick was to find a technique that would encourage this.

These problems not only affected Laurie and Marty: they were common to most players. The more you break your movements down into segments—mentally and physically—the more mechanical and awkward your playing becomes. Gradually I evolved a teaching method where I said less about the parts and asked the students to put more energy and body into both preparation and hitting the ball. They had to work harder and get more effort into each shot. But it was worth it. The balls they hit had more power, and they became less self-conscious and less concerned with technicalities. I began to see that this emphasis on whole body movement worked for every player and with each stroke.

These days, if you were to listen in on one of our practice sessions in Berkeley, you might hear me say: "Too much arm!" I don't mean, "Don't use your arm." What I *do* mean is, "Get your body behind your arm." Or, you might hear me say, "Don't run right at the ball!" I want the player to be able to use energy to get away from and behind the ball and then explode forward and hit with power.

This alive energetic approach, this eagerness and zest in chasing and hitting each ball—and the stimulating workout—are available to you. *Aerobic Tennis* will show you how to get more of *you* into each shot, how to concentrate on the physical aspects of the game and how to involve your whole body in everything you do on the court. Regardless of your age, skill or style, you will get the workout you've been looking for and improve your physical condition.

And what about winning? In one sense, you're a winner every time you practice or play a match this way. You have a good workout. You become more fit. You feel better and more alive. But in the real sense, you're also going to win. When you're in better shape, when you learn to hit the ball with your whole body, your shots will be harder to return and you're going to win more matches. □

# I. The Aerobic Method

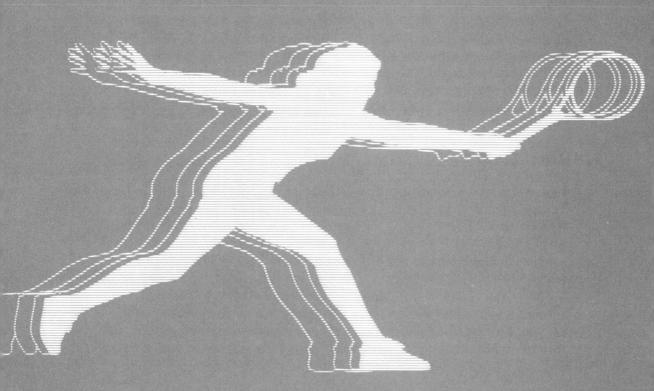

*"Tennis is a running game,"* one of the pros in Vail often yells at his students. That it is, but it's much more: it's a game for your whole body. Watch a top match on television. Follow one of the players during an entire point. Don't just watch the ball, but concentrate on the player's movements. You'll see quick starts, jumping, stretching, reaching, sprinting, sudden changes of direction—a total workout.

Now go down to your local courts and watch the "action." You won't see anywhere near the same level of physical intensity—not even a scaled-down version of a good workout. Something is holding these players back. They're agonizing over technique, or they're worried about how they look. All they're aware of is the net, the baseline, their opponent . . . so many difficult obstacles to overcome. All these restraints get in the way of good physical movement and the enjoyment of the game.

We're not going to over-emphasize the technical aspects of hitting the ball. There are already a number of excellent tennis books on technique (see bibliography, p. 184). And we're not going to ask you to copy anyone else's style. We're going to show you a method of playing tennis where you will involve your whole body in everything you do on the court, where you will take your present style, present skills and present strokes and make them more alive, vigorous and enjoyable.

## *The "Look"*

I was watching a new member hitting the ball a few years back at the Denver Tennis Club. After she played I went over to her and asked, "Are you from New Orleans?" She looked at me quizzically and told me she was. Then when I said, "And I bet your coach was Emmet Paré," she was really shocked. I explained that her backhand had given her away because all of Emmet's pupils hit the ball the same way.

Many teachers, and most tennis books, whether they say it or not, encourage you to imitate a look. In *Aerobic Tennis,* we encourage you to use your own present style, rhythm, skill and experience as a foundation—and then try to involve more of your body in each move you make. This will give you much more freedom of expression and you'll enjoy the game a lot more. There's no point in trying to look like a Chris Evert-Lloyd or a John McEnroe, because you won't. Besides, there's not one "look" that everyone should emulate.

## Be Yourself

On the following pages are drawings of different players hitting different shots. But these are only examples. You should work with your own unique style and natural abilities in developing sound strokes. A good example is Björn Borg, who grew up in a little town outside Stockholm. When he was about 12 years old, he was brought into a junior development program in Stockholm by a pro who was overhauling everyone's strokes. He was going to do the same to Borg's unorthodox style. When the head of the program, Davis Cup coach Lennart Bergelin, saw Borg play he said in effect, "Don't touch him. He has a flair and a natural rhythm that you mustn't tamper with." The result is evident. The way you hit the ball will depend upon a number of factors unique to *you*.

## The Feel

Often when I'm teaching, players will say, "I see what you mean." Actually, they have made a breakthrough, not in seeing, but in *feeling*. What they really mean is, "I feel what you mean." They finally *feel* the ball on the strings of the racket. Once you feel, for example, the power you can get on a volley with a short punching action and your body behind the ball, you'll wonder why in the world you needed a long elaborate swing. We want you to feel what it's like to hit a solid heavy ball, feel your knees bend, feel your body stretch, feel the racket relaxed in your hand before the hit, feel the lift . . . . I hope you'll be able to translate this book from the pages to your mind to muscle feeling.

## Conventional Teaching

How many times have you heard: "Get your racket back," or "Bend your knees," or "Straighten your elbow"? In conventional teaching, great emphasis is placed on the individual parts of the body. But almost all coaches have learned that when you direct your attention to a specific part of your body, you freeze up. You concentrate on the particular part so much you lose sight of the whole. When I'm ready to ski down the mountain and someone says, "Now remember to bend your knees . . .," I worry so much about my knees that I don't have a relaxed and enjoyable run.

## The Inner Game

W. Timothy Gallwey, in his best-selling book, *The Inner Game of Tennis,* provided the key for thousands of players to relax and play better tennis. In a sort of Zen Archery approach to the game, Gallwey advised the reader to " . . . just let it happen." This approach seemed to help many players who were nervous and uptight about their games. Amidst all the conventional books and teachers emphasizing technique, the individual parts of the body and imitation of other players, Gallwey came along and said, in essence: "Forget all those confusing details. Let your mind be clear, relax, don't overthink, just let it flow . . . watch the seams of the ball . . .," and voilà!–the jitters disappeared and people seemed to play better tennis.

## The Aerobic Method

Our method differs from both conventional teaching and the *Inner Game* approach. You're not going to over-analyze every move to the point of paralysis, but you're not going to surrender all conscious thought either. You're going to concentrate on involving your whole body in everything you do on the court, and on getting some good aerobic exercise. You're going to turn your body loose and run, stretch, leap and get a sweat up. You're going to get a better workout, thereby getting more fit. You're going to feel better, have more fun and therefore play more and better tennis. □

# II. Hitting the Ball

# Groundstrokes

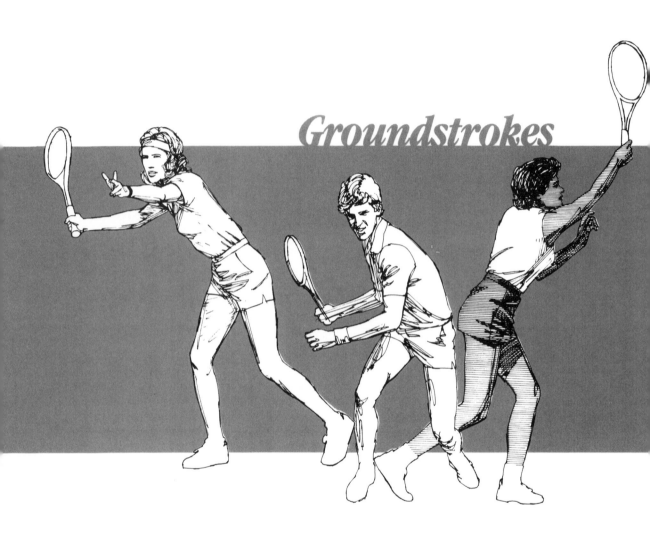

*Running, jumping, stretching, bending* . . . all of us can do these basic physical things. All of us have rhythm. And we don't lose our ability to perform these basic natural actions when we walk onto a tennis court. We are going to build on these familiar activities, recognizing that the skills needed to play good tennis are physical movements we have been making all our lives.

In hitting groundstrokes, just remember—there's nothing new or mysterious about the basic actions. In playing *Aerobic Tennis,* you're going to emphasize these moves, you're going to maximize effort. You're going to:

- Run as fast, as far, and as hard as possible.
- Get away from the ball so you can step into it.
- Stretch your muscles reaching out for the ball.
- Get your whole body into every move.
- Work up a sweat and get a great workout.

More balls will go into the court, they will be going much harder, you'll find yourself playing better, and you'll be having more fun. You'll be getting good aerobic exercise and increasing your total fitness.

I was in Palm Springs recently with the Cal team at a national intercollegiate tournament. We had finished working out and were passing behind some courts where we heard a lot of vocal and enthusiastic coaching going on. Though in different voices, the advice from all three coaches was the same: "Bend more . . . run more . . . reach farther . . . more body . . . more pivot . . . ." I peeked through the fence and saw three of the country's outstanding college coaches: Dennis Ralston of SMU, Glenn Bassett of UCLA and Dick Leach of USC working with their players.

How do you do what these coaches were asking for? You start thinking about getting your body into your groundstrokes so you will develop your agility, fitness and strength. For example, I was playing a match the other morning with a friend and I just wasn't having a good time. Then I thought, "Practice what you preach, coach." I decided to see how much I could run, turn, stretch and lunge. I started running harder, working to get farther away from the ball, started using my body, stretching and turning. Pretty soon I was sweating, having a good time and—not surprisingly—playing better.

# Dynamics of a Groundstroke

## Ready (to Move) Position

Too many players think of the ready position as a static one: clunk . . . feet planted . . . they're ready. Like pitching a tent. Instead of that, think of the ready position as a ready-*to-move* position.

Mentally, you're set. No ball is going to get past you, you're simply going to *run* every one down. Physically, you're set: to jump, to pivot, to change directions.

The ready position for every sport is about the same. For a shortstop, a defensive back before the snap, a guard in basketball: knees bent, legs shoulder-width apart, fanny down, weight forward on your toes. You are ready to *move*.

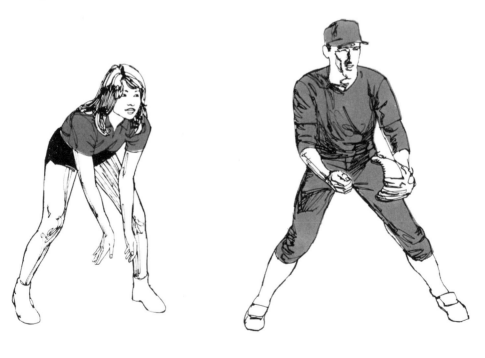

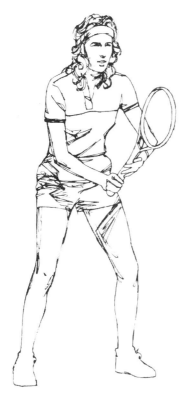

*Normal ready position*

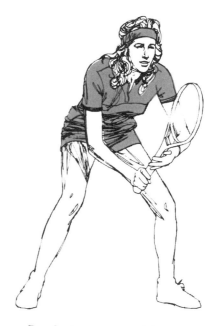

*Ready-**to-move** position*

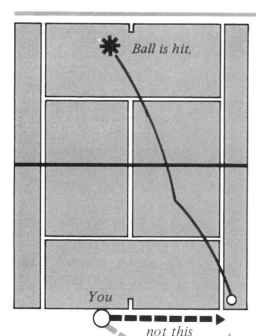

Ball is hit.

You

not this

but this

## *Footwork*

Your natural inclination is to get beside the ball and too close to it. How can you avoid that?

Once you see where the ball is going to land, don't run straight at it. Run behind it, then forward. You'll get more momentum and power that way and hit a better shot. You'll also run more and get a better workout.

Think of playing golf. The golfer addresses the ball. When he gets ready to hit it, he lays the club out to position himself *away* from the ball. The natural swing of his arms and body provides the power. Get away from the ball and give yourself some room to hit. Get your weight back on your rear foot so your weight can go forward into the shot.

You must cover the entire court. I often jokingly tell my students, "If you were the only one playing here, we'd only have to resurface a small part of the court." "Why?" they ask. "Because you just run up and down a two-foot path behind the baseline instead of moving up and back."

## Don't Just Bounce

Some pros tell you to "bounce—get on your toes." This isn't enough. Think of footwork as extending from your toes to hips to shoulders. Feel the energy go up your legs. Pick up your feet by using lift—use your thighs, hips and waist and see how different it feels, how much more fun it is and how much more weight you can put into each shot.

## "Knee Bone Connected to Your Thigh Bone"

This summer in Vail I worked with Kathy Carson, an exceptionally good player. Kathy had played on the Virginia Slims circuit and had hurt her knee but was now starting to play again. I was explaining to her the method of using her whole body in hitting the ball. I said, "Think of your footwork as a body function. It's not just getting on your toes and bouncing, but it's preparation and movement from your feet up to your shoulders." You should have seen her hitting the ball. It was phenomenal. She had an entirely different look, more confidence, more power and grace.

*Your Daily Vacation . . . I heard recently about a high-powered, hard-pressured executive who had taken up jogging to relieve his tension. He should have played tennis. When you're on the court you can't think about anything but hitting the ball. You don't have time to think about your problems. Everyone needs to take a little vacation every day.*

## *Don't Just Get Your Racket Back*

One of the most familiar phrases used in teaching tennis is "get your racket back," with the admonition that the earlier you get it back the better. This has been poorly explained. If you just get your racket back—only the racket and arm back— then only the racket and arm can come forward, giving you nothing but an arm hit.

*The racket is back, and that's all.*

There are three important points to remember here:

1. Don't just take your arm back, but have your entire body take the racket back. It's a *whole body* function.
2. As your racket head goes back, the wrist lays back. The arm and the racket are not locked straight, *nor are they ever* in the forehand. The elbow is relaxed and *bent* throughout the swing. Don't straighten your arm and swing wide to "get your racket back." Take your racket back with your arm, elbow and body—always in control and ready to begin your forward swing.

*Let your upper body take your racket back.*
*When you swing it will be with your whole body.*

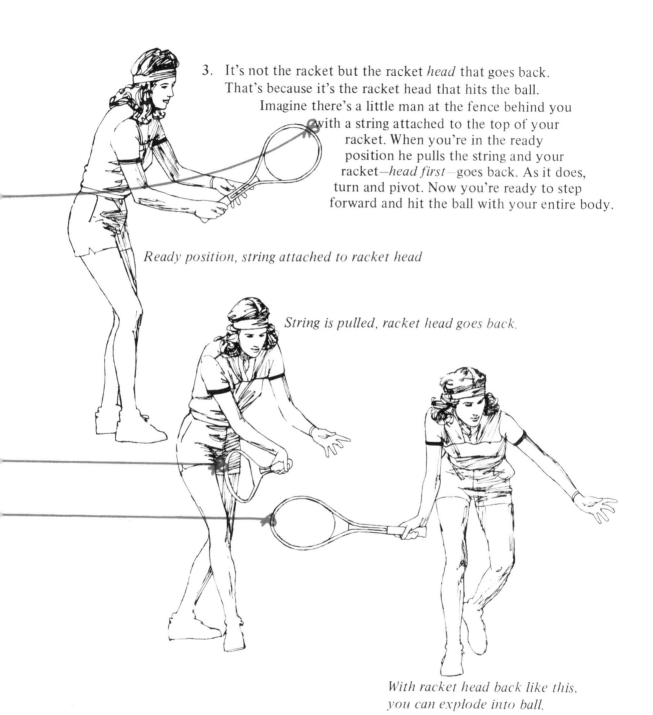

3. It's not the racket but the racket *head* that goes back. That's because it's the racket head that hits the ball. Imagine there's a little man at the fence behind you with a string attached to the top of your racket. When you're in the ready position he pulls the string and your racket—*head first*—goes back. As it does, turn and pivot. Now you're ready to step forward and hit the ball with your entire body.

*Ready position, string attached to racket head*

*String is pulled, racket head goes back.*

*With racket head back like this, you can explode into ball.*

## Don't Just "Get Sideways To the Net"

"Get sideways to the net" is another overworked and confusing phrase. You'll be locked into position with your weight going toward the side fence and straining to get the ball over the net. You'll only be using your arm to hit the ball. You *do* get sideways to the net, but it's part of the process of winding and unwinding (see below). What gets you in trouble is when you get stuck in that sideways position.

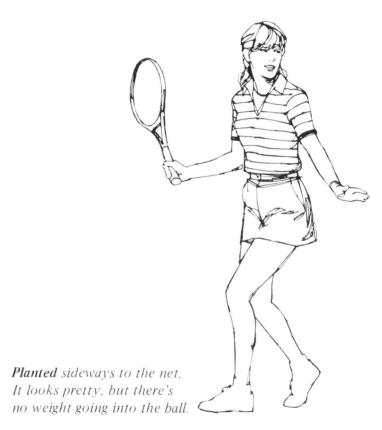

*Planted* *sideways to the net. It looks pretty, but there's no weight going into the ball.*

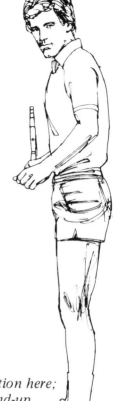

## Wind Up and Unwind

All hitting and throwing sports have a *wind-up*. The body winds up—and when it unwinds there is power. You coil, then uncoil. The more you turn your body, the more power you'll have when you unwind. You don't need a big arm swing; you're going to use your entire body in hitting the ball.

Get your hips, arms and fanny into it. Everything else—footwork, racket preparation, the hit and follow-through—is a development of this basic wind-up and unwind theme. Unwind naturally and rhythmically. Think of your body, arm and racket head as one unit, with the racket head leading the band.

*Not much action here; there's no wind-up.*

## More Than Meets the Eye

When you're trying to learn how to play tennis by watching a match, and you're just watching the ball, you're not really seeing how the shot is hit. You don't realize how much a good player has put into body preparation. It's like watching a football game. When you see an end catch a TD pass it looks so easy. He and the ball have somehow miraculously ended up at the same spot. But when you watch the instant replay you see him getting bumped at the line of scrimmage, faking and changing directions, then fighting off a defender to make that catch. It was anything but easy.

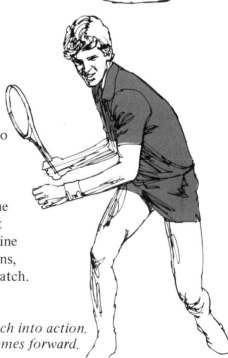

*Coiled position: body ready to launch into action. Everything goes back, everything comes forward.*

Likewise when you're watching a match, you're not aware of the effort and energy and struggle of the good players getting into position. When you see them they're perfectly set up to hit the ball and their strokes are flowing and beautiful. And you marvel . . . how did they do that? But if you watch from the very beginning you'll see the players struggling and running just to get into a position to hit the ball. It doesn't just happen.

## When to Start the Wind-Up

You start your wind-up as soon as your opponent hits. The speed at which you coil and uncoil will depend upon the speed of the oncoming ball. But it will also depend upon the quickness of your reflexes, your own rhythm, your own fitness. Just remember, wind up *early*.

## The Grip

*His body is behind the racket.*

The grip is crucial for a whole body hit, since this is where your body and the racket join forces. Your groundstroke grip must allow your body to absorb the shock of the hit. You get this strength by having the "meat" of your hand behind the racket at the hit. This gets your body behind it.

You'll notice that when you have a good grip, your body's behind the racket all the way through the stroke. When you have a bad grip your body is probably ahead of the racket at the point of impact.

## *Use Your Left Hand*

Tennis is not a one-handed game. You'll find the more you (right-handers) use your left hand, the more turn and therefore the more body you'll be getting into the forward swing.

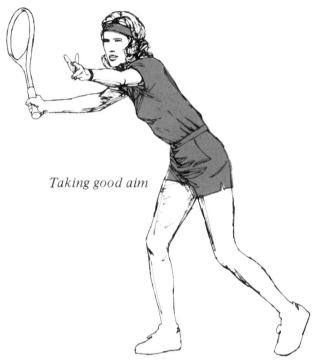

*Taking good aim*

*Left-Handers:*
*For simplicity our instructions are for right-handers. If you're left-handed, just reverse things when we say "left hand" or "right hand."*

Aiming your left hand at the oncoming ball helps you:
- Turn your shoulders.
- Track the ball.
- Measure your distance from the ball.
- Get the left side of your body engaged in the shot.

Don't let your left hand droop. Dropping the left hand and "standing sideways to the net" go hand in hand—like ham and eggs. If you do one, you almost inevitably do the other. This is probably the most common forehand groundstroke fault.

## *Teeter-Totter*

Your shoulders work like a teeter-totter. As you sit here reading this, drop your left shoulder as you would if you let your left arm "hang" while playing. What happens to the right shoulder? It raises. On the court this means that your right shoulder and racket, which you want down and below the ball—for the low-to-high effect—are way too high; you'll be hitting down and the ball will tend to go into the net. Keep your left hand up at ball level or above.

## *The Hit*

It's not really a "hit." You *hit* a nail, you *stroke* a groundstroke. A stroke is one continuous action, from ready position to follow-through. The hit is merely the point along the stroke where the racket meets the ball.

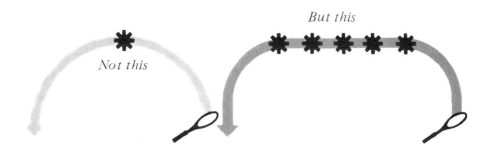

*But this*

*Not this*

When you paddle a canoe, you do not *hit* the water with your oar and expect the boat to travel. Your action is a long stroke through the water. Similarly, try to keep the racket on the ball as long as possible.

Now go for it! This is what you've been waiting for: the contact of the ball with the strings. Hit in front of you. Use that body. Whenever you have a chance to watch a good player, note how in the best shots, the player's body and racket work together. The racket looks like an extension of the body. Everything flows. With the weaker shots, you'll be aware of the isolated arm movements. The body is left out.

## *What About the Net?*

It's simple. Lift the ball to get it over the net. I often tell my students in Vail to look at the ski lift, which is directly behind the court. Your stroke starts low and ends high. To get the ball over the net you must start low and end high. If the ball goes long, your ski slope is too steep. If it goes into the net, your slope is too flat.

## *Up the Ski Lift*

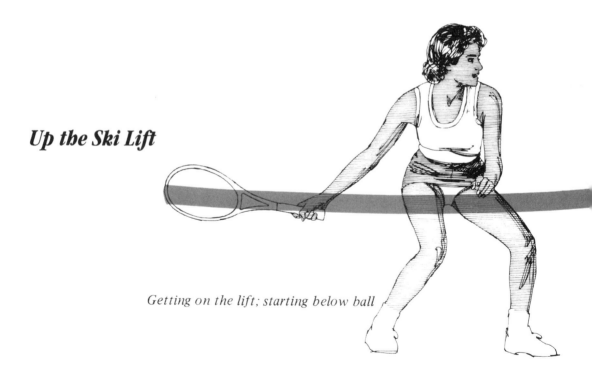

*Getting on the lift; starting below ball*

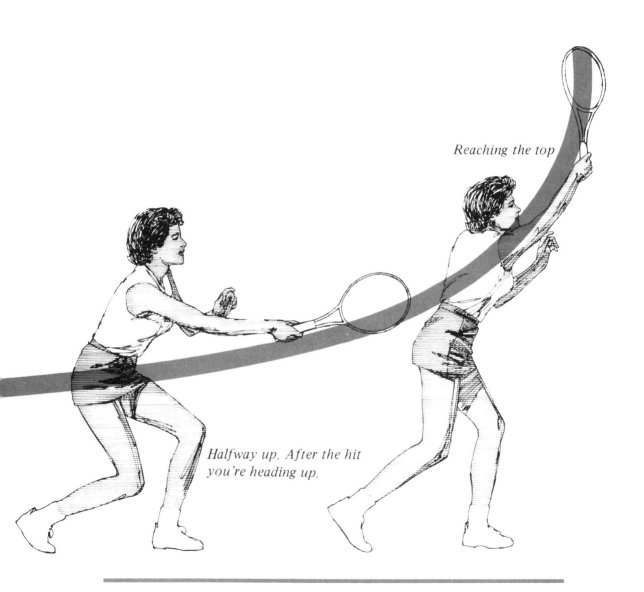

*Reaching the top*

*Halfway up. After the hit you're heading up.*

## *What If the Ball Doesn't Go Where I Want It To?*

The ball will go in the direction the racket face is pointing. If you want it to go cross-court, your racket face must be pointing in that direction.

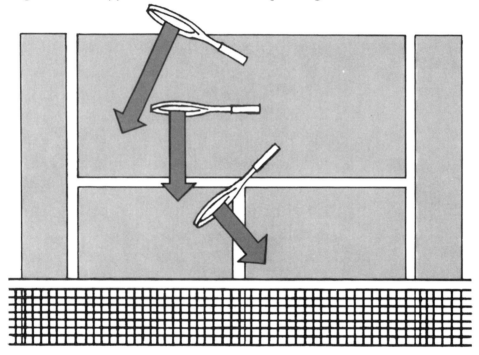

## *What About the Baseline?*

If your groundstrokes are sailing over the baseline, go back to emphasizing your low-to-high swing (the ski lift) — this will naturally generate topspin (see p. 102). This spin, along with a little help from gravity, will bring the ball down into the court.

## *Your Perfect Ending*

Stretch. Reach toward your target with everything: racket, shoulders, hips and knees. Your racket ends up at the top of the ski lift. Your weight is forward because you've pivoted after the hit. You'll be balanced and ready for the next ball.

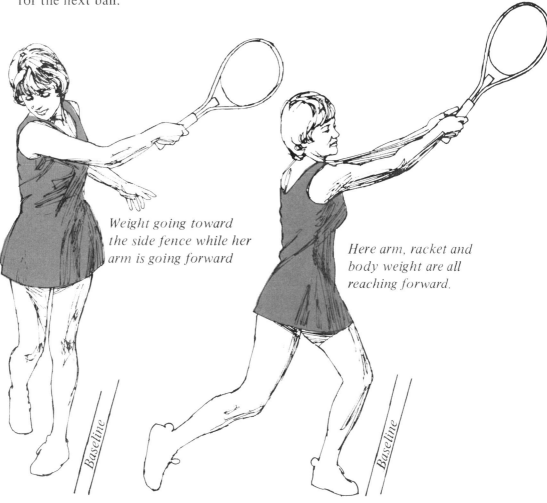

*Weight going toward the side fence while her arm is going forward*

*Here arm, racket and body weight are all reaching forward.*

*Baseline*

*Baseline*

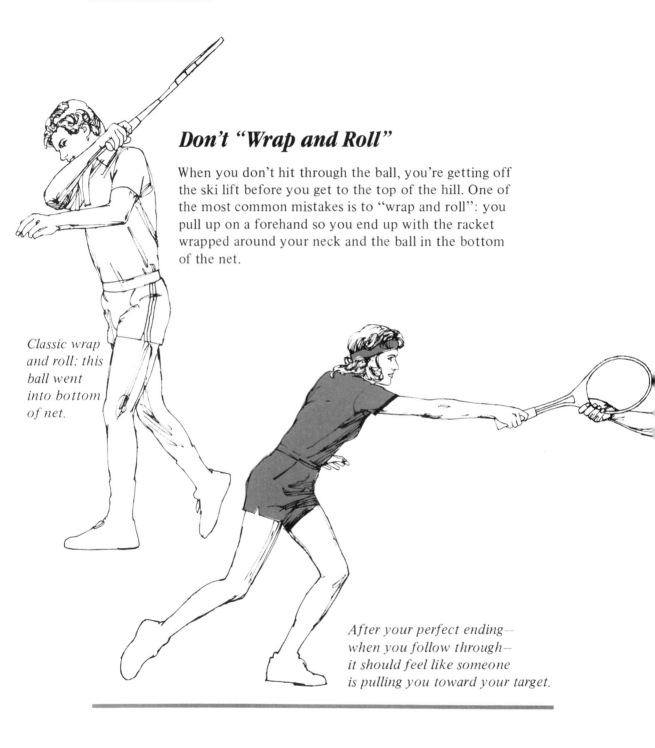

## Don't "Wrap and Roll"

When you don't hit through the ball, you're getting off the ski lift before you get to the top of the hill. One of the most common mistakes is to "wrap and roll": you pull up on a forehand so you end up with the racket wrapped around your neck and the ball in the bottom of the net.

*Classic wrap and roll; this ball went into bottom of net.*

*After your perfect ending— when you follow through— it should feel like someone is pulling you toward your target.*

# *The Backhand*

Don't ever think, "Oh no!" when you see that backhand coming. You can learn to enjoy it, as many players have in recent years, and you may discover a potent weapon. Many players actually have a better backhand than forehand because the body isn't in the way of the hitting arm. If you think about the concept of pivoting on the forehand, you'll see why the backhand—for some players—is easier. There's no body to get out of the way.

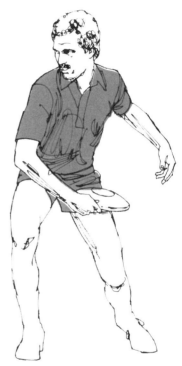

*The unwinding on a backhand is as simple as throwing a frisbee.*

## *Feet Frozen?*

Fear of the backhand is quickly translated into inaction from your feet up to your shoulders. Hustle to get behind the ball—just like you would on a forehand—so your movement will be forward. Other than a change in the grip, the basic dynamics of a backhand in our way of playing tennis are the same as a forehand: Winding up and unwinding, hitting through the ball, the racket going up the ski-lift and *through to the perfect ending.*

## *Knuckles Up*

To hit good backhands you need a good grip. You want to hit the ball in front of you, with your body and all its weight and power behind the hit. To do this, you must change your grip from the forehand position.

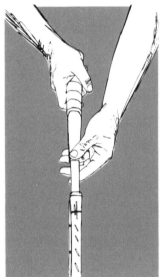 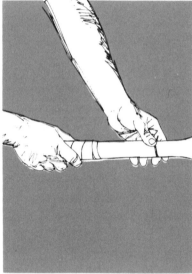 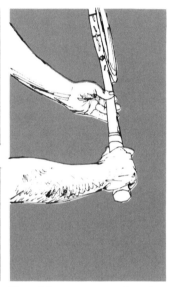

*Forehand grip*

*Transition: on its way to backhand*

*Knuckles up: completed backhand grip*

Don't try to make this change in the ready position—when your grip should be in neutral. But when you see the ball coming to your backhand, start your racket back (being carried by the left hand) and your grip will naturally rotate over the top. You should be able to see your knuckles. As a reminder, think: *Knuckles up.*

Your grip will vary depending upon the position of the ball. Don't let your grip dictate how you're going to hit the ball, but let the ball and its position dictate the grip.

# Two-Handed Backhand

Tennis is a two-handed game, unlike squash or racquetball where you just use one. There are two ways you can use the left hand in hitting backhands:

1. *In preparation:* You use your left hand to guide the racket in the backswing, but then release the racket and let one hand do the hitting. Use of the left hand this way—in *preparing* to hit a backhand:

   - Helps you change your grip, because it supports the racket.
   - Helps you turn and get power.
   - Keeps your racket head down and below the ball.
   - Helps you gauge where the racket head is in relation to the ball.

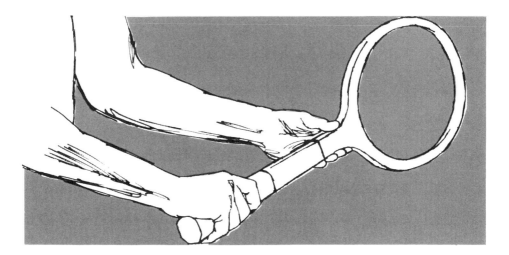

When the left hand is close to the head of the racket, you have a part of your body in close contact with the racket head and you know where it is in relation to your body. If your left arm stays fairly straight and down, then you know your racket head is down.

2. ***Throughout the stroke****:* The other use of the left hand in backhands is to use it throughout the entire stroke, including the hit.
   You've undoubtedly seen the great two-handed backhands of
   Jimmy Connors or Chris Evert-Lloyd. For some players, however,
   a two-handed backhand may feel restrictive because it's hard to hit
   backhand volleys and those wide balls. In general, two hands
   should be used by a player who finds it natural, or by one who
   can't hit a strong enough backhand with one hand. Otherwise,
   let go with your left hand when you start your forward swing.

*Two hands
with body =
plenty of power*

# *Word Pictures*

## *Hitting a Heavy Ball*

Bill Tilden was one of the first to use the term. It means you're hitting a ball at just the right moment, keeping it on the strings a long time and getting your weight behind it. The ball is "heavy" when your opponent hits it. One of the best examples of a "heavy ball" I can think of is Pancho Segura's forehand. I played Segura in a pro tournament in Monterey some years ago and later, when I was working in Los Angeles, would play against him in doubles in Pasadena every Monday. Pancho seems relaxed and loose when he hits the ball, but when it hits your strings you feel like you're hitting a shotput. It's so deep and heavy that it pushes you further back into the court. After about three balls, you're against the ropes—you're struggling just to get the ball back over the net, let alone move him around the court. All great shots in tennis are "heavy"—Segura's and Borg's forehands or Connors' backhand.

## *Hitting Through the Ball*

An expression frequently used, it means starting your stroke behind the ball and finishing your stroke with your racket pointing where you want the ball to go. You keep the ball on the strings as long as you can—sweeping, not batting the ball—and keep your racket in line with the flight of the ball. The word pictures "hitting a heavy ball" and "hitting through the ball" help you picture what it's like to hit the ball well.

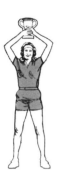

# *Tips—Groundstrokes*

1. Involve your entire body, all the way down to your toes. Don't muscle it, but let it flow.
2. Keep your stroke smooth—stroke through the ball.
3. Get set to hit the ball earlier than usual. This way you'll have more body in it.
4. Don't worry about hitting the ball long. Just stroke it up and over the net. Gravity and topspin will keep it in.

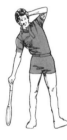

# *Trouble Shooting—Groundstrokes*

| *Trouble* | *Probable Reason* | *Try This* |
|---|---|---|
| ● ball sails over baseline | ● too much underspin (see pp. 100-103 on spin). <br> ● not enough follow-through | ● get racket & arm down and below ball in backswing <br> ● exaggerate follow-through up ski lift (see p. 26 ) |
| ● ball lands too short or into net | ● hitting down into ball or pulling up (wrap & roll) <br> ● racket face closing | ● bend legs, get under ball & stay with it <br> ● open racket face |
| ● poor ball placement | ● hitting too late | ● take ball earlier <br> ● keep racket face pointing to target |
| ● no pace; ball too weak | ● hitting only with arm; not enough body in shot | ● stay away from ball <br> ● move body into shot |

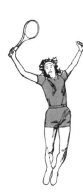

# *Fitness Goals—Groundstrokes*

1. *Turn* your entire body. Wind up as much as possible.
2. *Shift* weight to your rear leg, in the backswing, like a knee-bend.
3. *Explode* forward, thrust forward—with your legs.
4. *Reach* and *stretch* toward your target. ☐

# Volleys

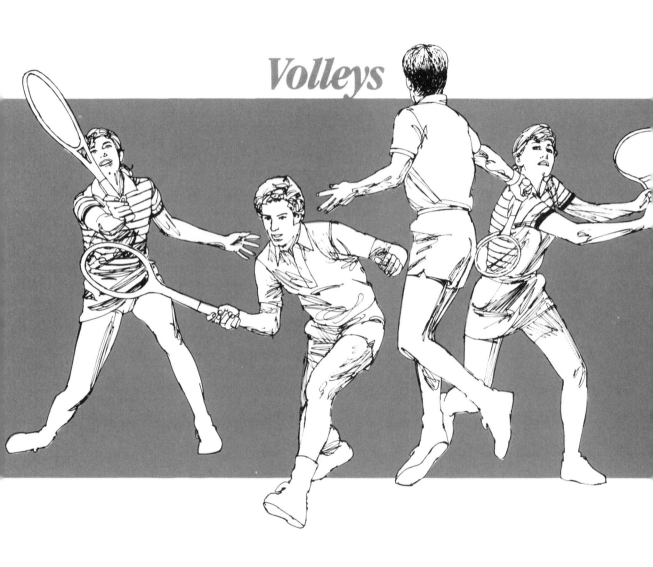

*When you come to the net,* the music changes. The tempo picks up. You twist and shout. Whereas in groundstrokes you have time to wind up and unwind and stretch your entire body, in volleys your actions are quicker and more spontaneous. You don't have time to line up every ball as you do on a groundstroke. You react, jump and attack with speed. You have to leap/dive/scramble at a moment's notice; this is part of the fun of volleying.

You may have heard that a volley is just a shorter version of a groundstroke. That's wrong; there's a world of difference between the two. When you think of the volley as a short groundstroke, you get into trouble. When you're up at the net, you're much closer to both your opponent and your target. You don't have time for a swing, so drop the groundstroke mentality.

## *Punch It*

A volley is a short, firm block of the ball. Tennis teachers often describe the volley as a short "punching" action without any further explanation. When you punch something you go directly toward it—very little backswing and very little follow-through. When you swing at something, there is a long sweeping motion. These are two entirely different actions. (Of course, the further you are from the net, the longer the volley action will be.)

With a volley, you don't *swing.* In fact, the shorter the stroke the better your volley. Some years ago, Rod Laver summed up the evolution of a good volley. He had just turned professional and the caliber of his opponents was much tougher. As greater demands were made on his playing, his volleys got better. He said, "I'm playing better because my volleys are better. My volleys are better because I swing less."

The volley is like the bunt in baseball. When a batter decides he is going to bunt the next pitch, rather than swing for the grandstands, the first thing he does is get the bat in front of his body. Then he changes his grip—holding the bat by his fingertips and not the palms of his hands; this gives him *feel.*

It's exactly the same in a volley. Once you realize the next shot will be a volley, bring the racket quickly in front of your body and hold it lightly in your fingers—not down in the palms. To help you visualize the short, compact action of the volley, think of catching a ball in your hand.

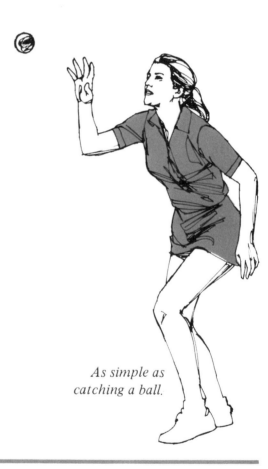

*As simple as catching a ball.*

## *Choke Up*

When you're learning to volley—not while playing—try choking up on your racket: Hold it high up on the handle, very close to the racket face. The closer your hand is to the racket face the easier it is to feel what the wrist is supposed to do. If you've been having trouble volleying this should help— it makes you identify your hand with the racket face. Once you get the feel of the hand and the racket face working together, stop choking up. Return to your normal grip.

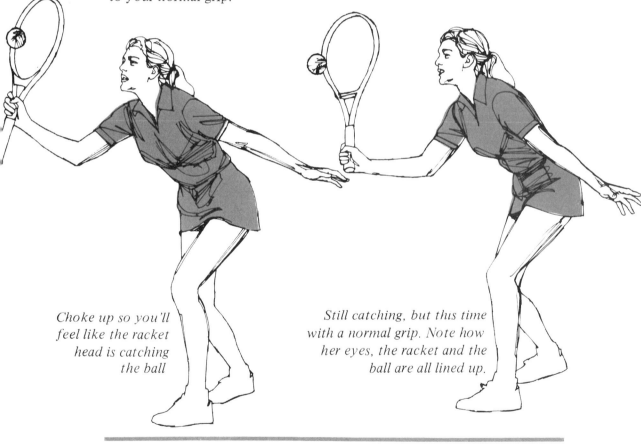

*Choke up so you'll feel like the racket head is catching the ball*

*Still catching, but this time with a normal grip. Note how her eyes, the racket and the ball are all lined up.*

# Dynamics of a Volley

## Ready (to Leap) Position

Right before your opponent hits the ball—regardless of where you are on the court—you come to a split-stop with legs bent, weight on toes, ready to jump in any direction. Lean forward and hold your racket so the head is up and out. Your ready position here is more crucial than on groundstrokes when you have more time to react.

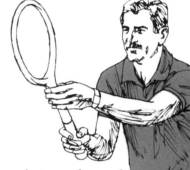

*Racket head up and out, ready to go forward*

## When to Come to the Net

Picture a traffic light:

- *Green light:* if your opponent hits a short ball that bounces inside your service line, come into the net.
- *Yellow light:* if it's behind the service line, but more than two yards from the baseline, be careful about going in.
- *Red light:* if it's within two yards of the baseline, don't come in.

## *"X" Does Not Mark the Spot*

Each player, regardless of ability, will have to make a decision on each point about where to stand. There is no one position that is good for every ball. Many of my students get frustrated with me because I don't put an "x" on the court showing where they should stand for every volley. By way of explaining that here "x" does *not* mark the spot, I tell them that proper net position will depend upon several factors:

- Their opponent's position.
- Their opponent's shot.
- Their own shot.
- Their own speed and height.

Lately, I've been using the concept of a circle to describe to students where to stand at the net. There isn't just one position for a volley, as many players think.

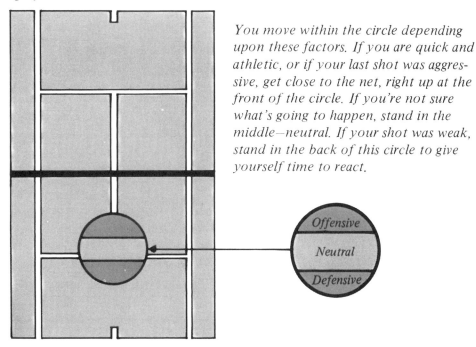

*You move within the circle depending upon these factors. If you are quick and athletic, or if your last shot was aggressive, get close to the net, right up at the front of the circle. If you're not sure what's going to happen, stand in the middle—neutral. If your shot was weak, stand in the back of this circle to give yourself time to react.*

## Short Steps

On groundstrokes, you have more time to get set, to dig in. On a volley, you don't—you must move quickly with short steps. On groundstrokes, because you can generally set up the shot, your weight will be going into the shot—toward the net. On a volley, the speed of the oncoming shot may not leave you time for anything more than a step, a short jump to the side, a stretch or a leap.

*Step Across:* you should always try to step from your left foot on a forehand and your right foot on a backhand. Stepping across like this will give you balance, reach and a solid foundation to hit from.

## How Low Can You Go?

To get more of a workout on the volley, get down as low as you can and push forward toward your target with thrust. Feel your legs pushing you, the racket and the ball. Pick up your feet. Move. Be aggressive. You should be able to *hear* your forward foot hitting the ground. If you do, you know you're transferring your weight.

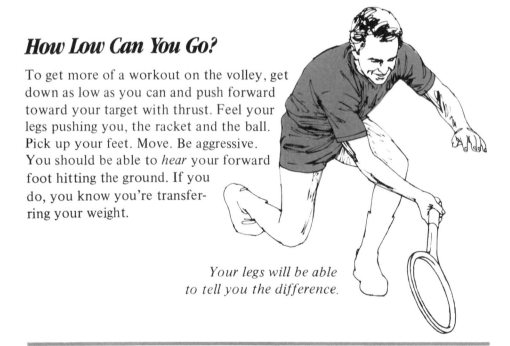

*Your legs will be able to tell you the difference.*

## The Grip

Hold the racket up and in front of your body. The grip is relaxed so that it is adjustable—the best grip for a low volley will be quite different from one for a high volley. The left hand is on the upper part of the racket handle while the right hand grips the handle.

Wilmer Allison, a former national champion in the '30's and a superb volleyer, advocated a different grip for every volley. His hands and wrists were relaxed enough before hitting the volley that he could make subtle adjustments in the racket face for each shot. Don't grab hold of your racket and say, "This is the grip I'm going to use for the rest of the day." Stay flexible.

## The Fear Factor

Many players are afraid of getting hit in the face when they're up at the net. When I have a pupil who has this fear, I have him stand very close to the net without his racket. I begin by throwing a ball very easily right at his face and ask him to reach out with his hitting hand and catch the ball. Then I start throwing the balls faster. Next, he picks up his racket, choking up on it, and again I pitch the balls. This time he blocks the balls with his racket directly back to me. When he gets comfortable doing this, I have him grab the racket by the handle, in a normal playing position.

*No fear here because the racket's in front of your face*

If you have a fear of being hit in the face, practice this routine with your partner. Try to *see* the ball through the racket strings. This will help you get the racket in front of your body and also make you get down to the shot. Line up your *head*, the *racket* and the *ball*.

## Step Aside? Never!

You may often be undecided about how to handle a ball coming straight at you at the net. Always try to step forward—keeping your racket between your face and the ball—and always try to use your forehand. Don't step aside; this will tempt you to swing—which you don't want to do here.

## Use Both Hands

Reach out with your left hand as well as the right. The left hand actually carries the racket, while the right hand is relaxed and just goes along for the ride. When you start your forward swing, the right hand takes over and you punch the ball.

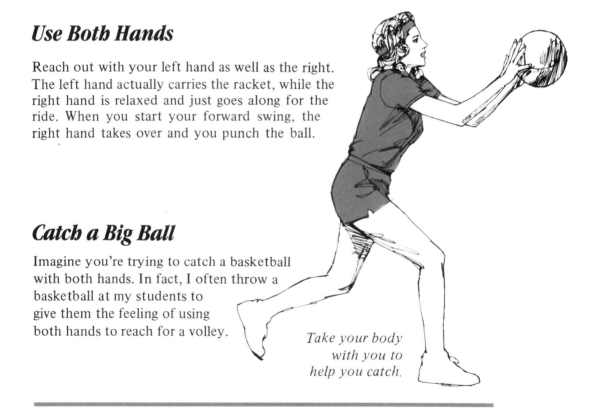

## Catch a Big Ball

Imagine you're trying to catch a basketball with both hands. In fact, I often throw a basketball at my students to give them the feeling of using both hands to reach for a volley.

*Take your body with you to help you catch.*

Reaching to catch that imaginary ball will make you do the following things naturally, without having to think about them:

- Turn your shoulders.
- Wind and unwind from the hips.
- Step forward.
- Get your weight underneath the ball.

Just catch that ball and see how these will fall in place.

## Pick a Spot and Go for It

Once you've decided where to hit the ball, don't look at your opponent and don't look at the spot where you want the ball to go. This will take your mind off watching the ball and following through. When you've picked a spot, don't change your mind—no guessing. Go for it.

## No Big Swing

How can I hit the ball hard without swinging? Don't worry. Remember the two factors that distinguish a volley from a groundstroke:

- The ball coming at you has much more power because you're closer to your opponent. (It loses speed the farther into your court it travels.)
- You are closer to your target and therefore don't need to swing as hard.

*Burning Rackets . . . Bill Tilden, the great champion of the 1920's, would sometimes play badly and lose. He'd come home depressed and distraught and swear he'd never play again. At night he'd dream of burning rackets. But the next morning he'd be out there playing tennis again. He'd hit the ball in the middle of the strings and have the indescribable thrill of the gut and ball connecting just right. He'd get a tremendous lift and get so excited that he'd wonder how he ever thought of giving up tennis.*

## *The Power of a Punch*

Here are two ways to practice a short swing:

- *By yourself:* Stand 10 to 12 feet from a backboard and try to rally. If your swing is too long the rally will be quite short, as the ball will go past you.

- *With a partner:* Both of you stand 8 to 10 feet away from the net and try to rally. Keep the ball off the ground. Again, if your swing is too big, you will have a short rally.

Once you begin to feel the power of the short punching action you get with this method, your whole conception of volleying and net play will change radically. You'll begin to enjoy volleying. You'll no longer feel like you're in a cage with too little time and space to react. You'll find there is time to change your grip, and to hit the ball with speed and direction.

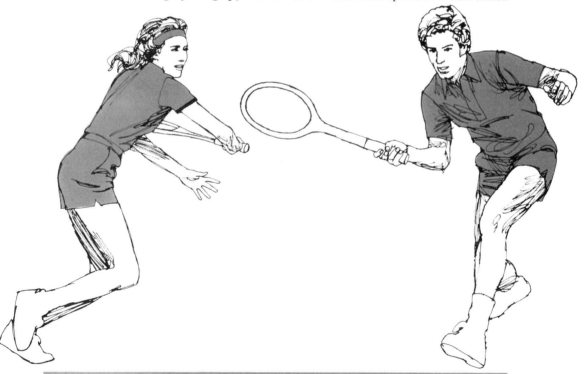

## *Short and Sweet*

Just before hitting, squeeze the racket strongly. Then give the ball a short powerful thrust slightly down through the ball towards the target. No big backswing—just short and sweet.

## *Spin*

There are two kinds of volleys—those above the net level and those below.

- *Above net level:* Here spin is of little concern. Just attack the ball. Your objective is to direct the ball down into the court. Pick a spot and go for it.
- *Below net level:* The real test of good volleying is how you handle a volley below net level. You have to understand spin to handle these balls effectively. You take the racket head back slightly above the ball, push it down and through the ball so that the ball has underspin. This lifts it over the net and gives it direction and pace. The main thrust is still through, not down.

  To teach this I often have a student stand 2 to 3 yards behind the net. I place a teaching basket on my service line and ask the student to punch volleys *into* the basket. Trying to do this he or she will learn to lift the ball over the side of the basket by underspin. If you don't have a teaching basket, put a cardboard box on a bench.

## *Be Decisive*

The volley is a natural follow-up to an effective serve or groundstroke. If you can't hit good volleys, you won't have an effective game plan. Most tennis strategy is geared to giving you a simple volley at the net. If you can't put the ball away, you will be frustrated time and again when points that should have been yours go to your opponent, like a basketball team executing a flawless play only to have the wide-open player miss an easy lay-up.

When you have an easy volley, be aggressive—go for it. Nothing is worse than having the volley that should have been a winner come back over your head because you were too tentative in punching it.

## *The Reluctant Volleyer*

When you're a beginner you're reluctant to go to the net. You feel awkward because it's strange and new. There is nothing a pro or a book can do to overcome this reluctance. You are the only one that can do it, and you can do so the next time you play. Come to the net behind your serve. Take a short ball and come to the net. Take that high floating groundstroke, volley it and come to the net. Once you get there, your competitive desire to hit the ball and cover the court will take over.

Even experienced players don't come to the net as often as they should because they have found a "comfort zone" in the back court. They feel they have a good chance to return every ball. They forget the threat and pressure their opponent feels by their mere presence at the net. Face it, you're going to miss some balls and some will go past you. But in the long run the percentages for winning are with you—the volleyer. Punching a few volleys to the open court will have you addicted to net play in no time. *Aerobic Tennis* is designed to get you to the net, to give you these exciting athletic experiences.

*Up at the net, attacking a return*

## Be Creative

You'll want to hit most volleys in hard, flat punches to the baseline, but if your opponent is dug in on the baseline, a soft angled shot just over the net may win the point easily. This is where the artist in you can come out. The volley is where you can test your ability to touch and feel the ball.

## Cool-Hand Mac

Bud Collins, who announced the 1982 Wimbledon championships, calls John McEnroe "the kid with the asbestos hands." He's talking about how McEnroe, with an almost magical touch, can take the fire out of a sizzling shot. When he's at the net and someone blasts the ball at him, he'll take the speed out of it and hit a delicate half-volley or drop-volley right over the net with a feathery touch. The ball will come to him at 90 mph and he'll change the speed to 20 mph.

# Backhand Volley

No shot in tennis is more aggravating than a poorly hit backhand volley. Any bad habits of your backhand groundstroke are carried over and magnified because here the ball is coming to you faster. To handle this shot well, you must hit it earlier, firmer, crisper and with less spin and more body. A tall order? Not really, if you remember the two important points of a good forehand volley—even more crucial here:

1. Use of the left hand. This allows you to relax the right hand, making your hand and wrist more flexible so you can change your grip.

2. Need for your body to be behind the racket and ball at the hit. If you do both these things, many of the most common backhand volleying problems will disappear.

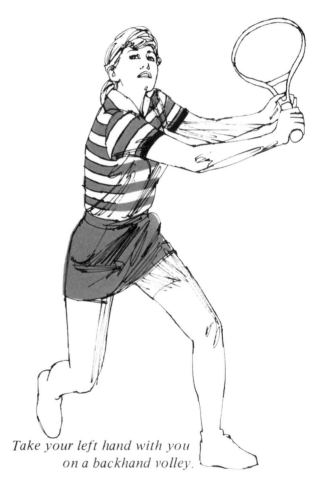

*Take your left hand with you on a backhand volley.*

## Karate Chop

Changing your grip allows you to hit the ball in front and your body is there to give support. It's like a karate chop.

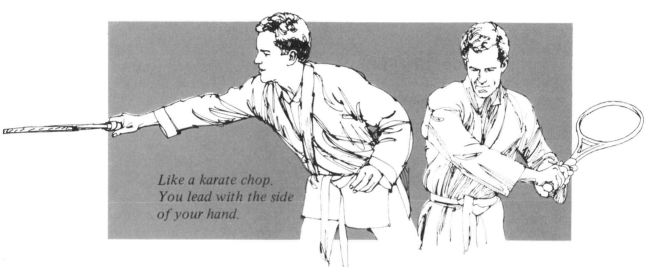

*Like a karate chop.*
*You lead with the side*
*of your hand.*

## Frozen at the Net?

Are you afraid of a backhand volley? You don't want the ball to come to your backhand, so you have a forehand state of mind and a forehand grip. Your grip is not in neutral. Then when the ball comes to your backhand, you're not only scared but surprised and you grab the handle harder and can't change your grip in time.

If you *do* have this problem, try to keep in a neutral state of mind at the net. After all, there's a 50-50 chance it *will* be a backhand. Keep your neutral grip. Look for that backhand, change your grip when you see it coming, and think of it as a chance to reach and punch the ball aggressively.

*The principles involved in hitting a backhand volley are basically the same as in the forehand volley: using the left hand, stepping forward, a short punch at the ball, etc. The major adjustment you make is the grip.*

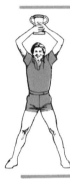

# *Tips*—*Volleys*

1. *Spring* forward.
2. *Hear* your footwork.
3. *Line up* your head, the racket and ball.

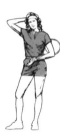

# *Trouble Shooting*—*Volleys*

| *Trouble* | *Probable Reason* | *Try This* |
|---|---|---|
| ●ball too long | ●too much swing, not enough punch | ●hit ball in front<br>●shorter punch |
| ●ball too short or into net | ●you're not under ball<br>●racket face closed | ●bend knees, get down<br>●more underspin |
| ●poor ball placement | ●not adjusting grip<br>●you're muscling it<br>●tight hands & wrists | ●relax hands & wrists<br>●more press-forward, less swing & hit |

# *Fitness Goals—Volleys*

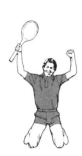

1. *Sprint* to your volleying position.
2. *Push* forward hard with your back leg.
3. *How low* can you go? Bend down for the low balls.
4. *Squeeze* racket strongly just before hit.
5. *Reach* for the ball with strength—direct it where you want it to go.☐

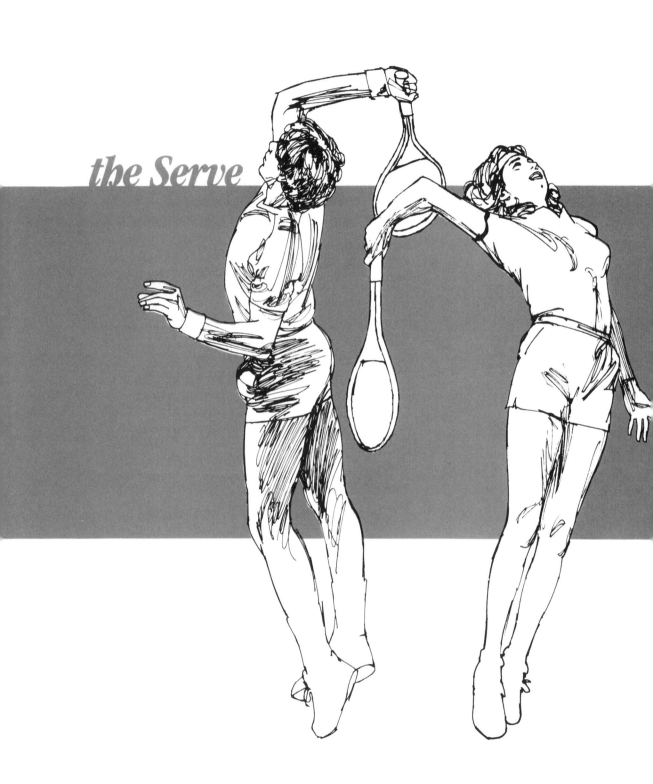

*the Serve*

*In every tennis clinic,* the mere statement, "Now let's hit a few serves," causes general consternation and even panic. It's like being called upon in class when you don't have the answer. A once enthusiastic class of 15 eager groundstrokers quickly shrinks to three reluctant servers with the rest of the class huddled near the fence.

Why do so many people get stage fright when serving? Probably because of the two distinct actions required: tossing the ball into the air, and then hitting it. Tennis is one of the few sports (volleyball is another) where you have to both throw the ball and hit it in the same motion. In golf, the ball is stationary; in baseball, the ball is pitched to you; in basketball and football, you're either catching it or throwing it. You don't have to both put the ball in motion and then hit it.

Hitting a serve needn't be intimidating. In fact, it's one of the most exciting and stimulating chances to reach and stretch that you'll find in sports. If you have ever thrown a ball, you have already performed many of the movements needed for an effective serve.

Throughout our discussion of serving, keep reminding yourself that the racket is an extension of your body, and at the point where the ball makes contact with the racket, it's your *entire body,* and not merely your wrist and forearm, that makes the ball travel. Keep this mental picture vivid in your mind and it will help eliminate confusion.

Think of the good serves you have seen; there is an exuberance in the hit. The player wasn't tense or timid or scared, but rather, was positive and eager about serving. If you find yourself getting tense, try holding a picture of a dynamic server in your mind.

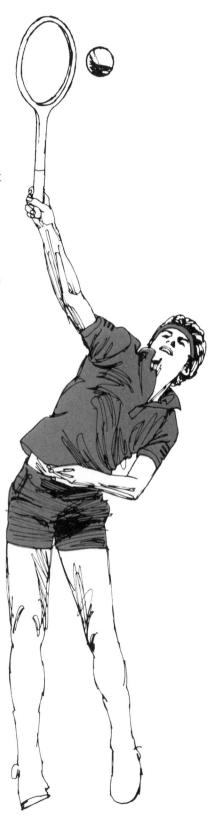

In 1963, I was playing in the finals of a tournament in Denver, and before the match had been watching Ile Nastase's powerful serves at Forest Hills. He was throwing the ball up high and in front and getting all his body into the serve. I tried retaining this vivid picture in my mind and it greatly improved my serve. Picturing a vigorous exploding serve will help overcome timidity and nervousness.

## Paralysis by Analysis

In teaching the serve, tennis pros generally go to one or the other extreme. They either tell you that the action of the serving arm is like throwing a ball and leave it at that, or they give you a paralyzing series of explanations analyzing and dissecting every angle.

The first method fails because serving is more than just throwing. There's also the toss and the coordination of the two. The second method fails because it makes learning to serve seem hopelessly complicated.

*No holding back here*

# Dynamics of a Serve

## Turn Your Brain Off

On a serve, you start from a standing, stationary position. It's up to you to set the ball in motion. When someone hits a groundstroke at you, the ball has its own motion and all you have to do is react. With a serve you must initiate the action. Here's the time to turn your brain off and let your body take over; it's more important here than almost anywhere else.

## Torque and Thrust

Line up your feet so you will get power two ways; from:

- Turning your shoulders (torque).
- Propelling your body forward through the hit (thrust).

You need to combine the two—torque and thrust—to get full power into the serve.

To illustrate this when teaching, I ask the student to face the right side fence and serve. If the serve *does* go in, the ball has very little power because the player has torque, but no forward motion. Then I ask the student to face the net, feet along the baseline, and serve. Here the server has plenty of thrust, but no torque. This serve will have no spin.

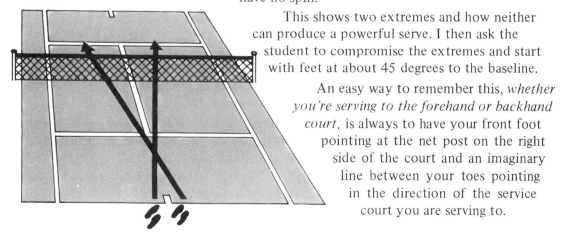

This shows two extremes and how neither can produce a powerful serve. I then ask the student to compromise the extremes and start with feet at about 45 degrees to the baseline.

An easy way to remember this, *whether you're serving to the forehand or backhand court,* is always to have your front foot pointing at the net post on the right side of the court and an imaginary line between your toes pointing in the direction of the service court you are serving to.

# Getting Started

Are you tentative about starting the service motion? To overcome this try starting out with your weight on the front foot and then point your racket at your opponent. You have to start somewhere and this gets things going. If you watch Martina Navratilova serve, you'll see her pointing her racket *at* her opponent. This gets her weight up and forward, gets her aiming in the right direction and allows her to rhythmically drop her arms and shift her weight to the rear foot. (It would obviously be intimidating to have Martina point her racket at you. You know she's concentrating, she's tuned in, and a cannonball serve is on its way.) In 1982, Jimmy Connors started pointing his racket and his serves were more powerful than ever. If you have trouble starting your serve, think of these three things:

● Weight forward.

● Point your racket.

● Let your arms drop.

# Rhythm

You have your own rhythm, your own music, unlike anyone else's. You may drop your arm several times before you toss the ball. John McEnroe does this and many baseball pitchers do it too. Once lined up, Jimmy Connors dribbles the ball six times and swings his arm loosely back and down.

# The Serving Grip

Start your serve by holding your racket in the forehand grip. Don't try a weird or uncomfortable position. To get the most power on your serve, your objective is to free your wrist. To do this hold the racket below the normal grip.

Many players spend years of their otherwise enjoyable tennis lives struggling with a modified backhand grip—in the hopes of adding spin to the ball. This generally gives them a brush *around* the ball—hence no power and lots of frustration.

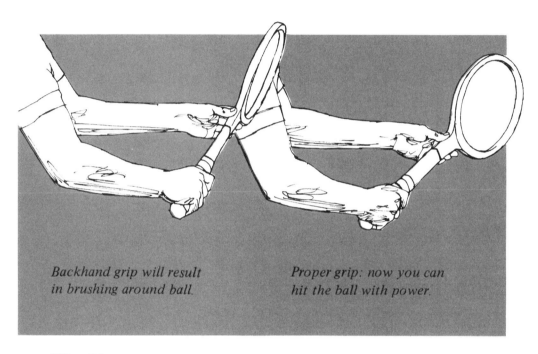

*Backhand grip will result in brushing around ball.*

*Proper grip: now you can hit the ball with power.*

## *The Toss*

"Toss" or "throw" are actually misleading terms. What you really want to do is *lay* or *place* the ball up in the air. (However, to avoid confusion, we'll say "toss.") When I'm teaching someone with an erratic toss, I'll often ask him to imagine that he's in a room and someone comes in, marks an "x" on the ceiling and says, "I'll give you $50 each time you can toss the ball and hit that mark." He'll invariably reach as high as possible toward the "x" with his arm rather than pitching the ball from waist height.

## The Tossing Arm

The simple objective of the toss? Getting the ball *high enough* to give your racket arm room to hit, and getting the ball far enough *in front* of you so your body will be *behind* the serve rather than under it. Put more than the wrist behind the toss. Release the ball when the tossing arm is fully extended.

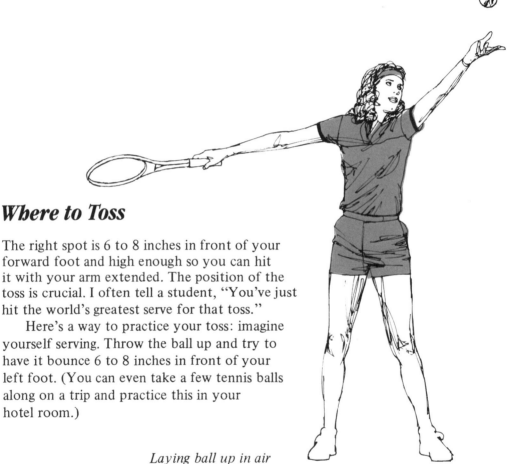

## Where to Toss

The right spot is 6 to 8 inches in front of your forward foot and high enough so you can hit it with your arm extended. The position of the toss is crucial. I often tell a student, "You've just hit the world's greatest serve for that toss."

Here's a way to practice your toss: imagine yourself serving. Throw the ball up and try to have it bounce 6 to 8 inches in front of your left foot. (You can even take a few tennis balls along on a trip and practice this in your hotel room.)

*Laying ball up in air*

Regardless of how much you practice, the heat of the battle may make you toss the ball in the wrong spot. If you do, don't hit it. Don't be self-conscious. Ken Rosewall wasn't: In the early '70's, Rosewall and Rod Laver were playing in the finals of World Championship Tennis for the largest prize money up to that time. During the course of the match, Rosewall threw the ball up and caught it instead of hitting it 37 times. He went on to win the match and didn't seem a bit embarassed.

## *The Magic Spot*

All of us would love to have the ball placed in the right spot and then held there for us to hit it. The closest we can come to this is to hit the ball at its most still point—that magic spot when the ball stops going up and starts coming down. To a beginner it seems as if a ball is either sailing up or falling rapidly. But the more you practice your toss and watch the ball, the easier it will be to identify that place where the ball is almost stationary.

*The magic spot: when the ball appears still*

## *Down Together—Up Together (and More)*

This is a fairly common description of the motion of your arms during the serve, but it's not quite accurate. The motion is actually *down together – back together – up together – forward together.* But for simplicity's sake, we'll also use the shorter term.

While the tossing arm is doing its job, what is the racket arm doing? Relaxing and falling back and up toward the throwing position. It's like a pendulum—no muscle is needed or desired. The looser here the better.

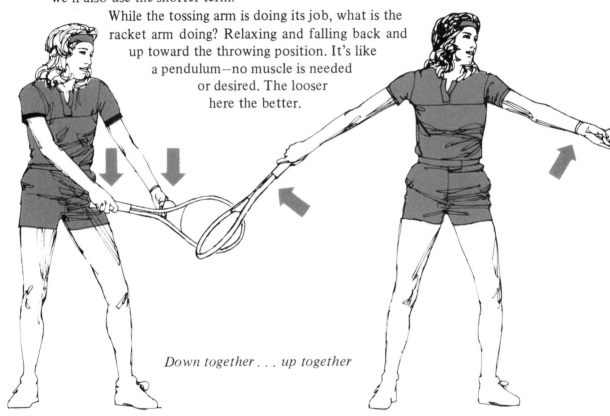

*Down together . . . up together*

## *The Hit*

Don't think of hitting. Think of *throwing* the racket with your whole body behind it to the spot where you want the ball to go. When Bill Tilden was teaching, he used to keep an old racket around and hand it to his student,

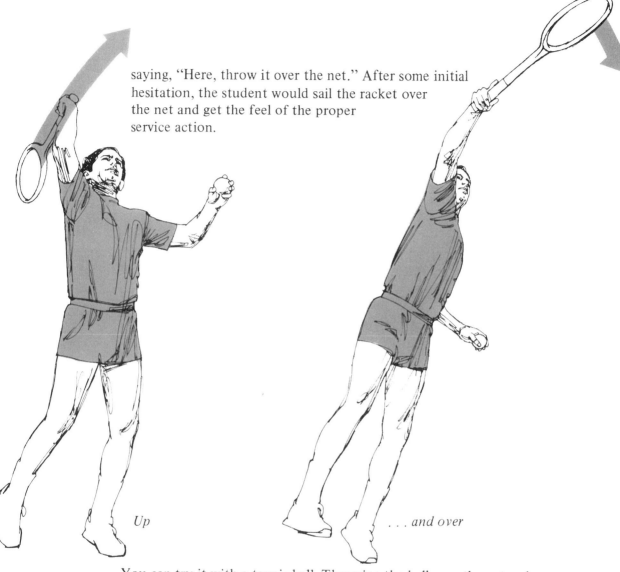

saying, "Here, throw it over the net." After some initial
hesitation, the student would sail the racket over
the net and get the feel of the proper
service action.

*Up*

*. . . and over*

You can try it with a tennis ball. Throwing the ball over the net and
thinking of it as serving gives you the feel of a free-flowing action. After
you've done this a few times, grab your racket and a half dozen balls and
go out on an empty practice court and try some serves. Throw your racket
through the ball just as you threw the tennis ball across the net. Remember
the ski lift (see p. 26)? Feel those strings going up and through the ball;
this will give you topspin.

## *On the Nose*

Chet Murphy, the tennis pro at the Broadmoor Hotel in Colorado Springs, uses a helpful word-picture when teaching serves. "Picture a face on the ball," Chet will say, and then he'll proceed to demonstrate with some serves. He'll hit one that goes long. "That ball was hit on the chin." Then one goes into the net. "That one was hit on the forehead." Or if the ball goes to the left, it was hit on the right ear, etc. Then he'll say, "Now I'm going to hit this one on the nose," and the ball will go into the court.

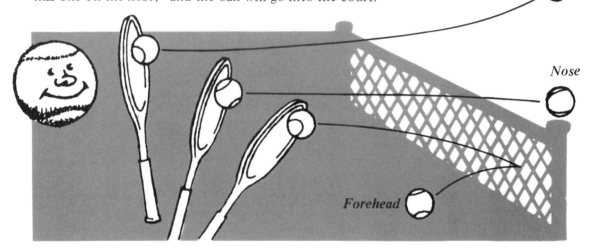

*Chin*

*Nose*

*Forehead*

## *Perfect Ending*

Beginning players will often slight the follow-through because they are so happy to have hit the ball. They breathe a sigh of relief. "Whew, at least I didn't whiff it."

For the nervous player—whether beginning or advanced—there is a great tendency to rush on all strokes and especially on the serve. Rush the toss, rush the hit and forget the follow-through. It's like that little snowball of mistakes rolling down the hill—it soon becomes an avalanche. We are so overly concerned with the return that we don't complete the stroke. We prematurely cut off a very important element of the serve. Stay with the stroke until it's completed. If you hit a solid heavy ball, there may not be a return.

A good follow-through will give spin, depth and pace to your serve. The body is reaching in the direction of the ball and is in a position to follow through. Let it go. Let your *whole body* hit the serve.

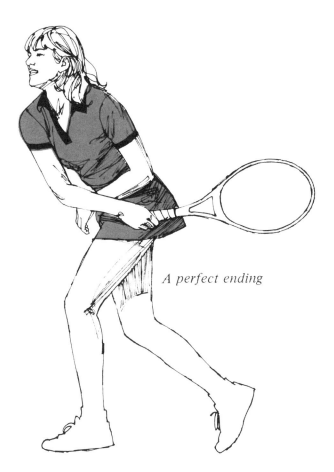

*A perfect ending*

Our players at Cal spend some time each week practicing serves—with no one returning. This way they can emphasize their follow-through, because they're not worrying about an opponent returning their serves. If you're having trouble with your serve, it will often be due to an incomplete or cramped follow-through. Try practicing with a basket of balls and no opponent.

## After the Perfect Ending

Remember, the serve *starts* the ball in motion. Even if you hit a good one, be ready and eager for the ball to come back. Your follow-through—your perfect ending—will have pulled you across the baseline. Bounce back to the baseline unless you're following your serve to the net.

*Sprint to the net after your perfect ending.*

## That Scary Second Serve

If you've faulted on your first serve, your tendency is to baby the second one. Get your body just as involved in the second serve as the first. Redirect your racket so that you hit up into the ball, giving it more torque and therefore more spin and margin over the net.

## *Foot Faults*

"Why don't you follow through on your serve?" I ask players at Vail. They'll say, "We can't end up in the court—that's a foot fault." They think there's an invisible barrier along the baseline. I keep reminding players that as long as the ball is hit *before* their foot crosses the baseline, there's no foot fault. *Do* follow through. Once you've hit the ball, swing forward with your hitting side into the court—it will give your serve much more power. Then use some energy to hop back to the baseline. Think: *follow-through—swing forward—hop back.*

## *Practicing Alone*

When you're practicing your serve alone, how do you tell if you're increasing your power and accuracy? Here are some suggestions:

- Note how high up on the opposite fence your ball is hitting. Try to make each succeeding serve hit up higher. You'll find yourself reaching up higher, getting your weight into it and developing more power.
- Place a target—a towel, for example—in the corner of the court and try to hit it. Them move the towel to the center of the service court. Often the most effective serve will be directly at your opponent.
- See how far into the court your follow-through leg ends up. The farther in, the more body you'll have put into the hit and the closer you'll be to the net. This is extremely important in doubles when you must get in behind your serve.

## *Everyone's Nervous*

Harry Hopman, the famous Davis Cup coach, always advised his players to receive serves when they won the toss at the beginning of a match. Even Davis Cup players are nervous serving—especially at the start of a match. He wanted his players to play a game receiving serves to loosen up before they had to serve.

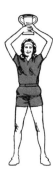

# *Tips*—*Serve*

If you're still having trouble with your serve, try one of these:

1. Forget the hit and concentrate on the toss:
   Stretch the tossing arm up, pushing the ball into the air.
   Get the ball forward.
   Get the ball high enough.

2. Keep a mental image of a dynamic server in your mind.

3. Slow down. Find your own rhythm. Line up correctly. Bounce the ball. Swing your arms back and forth.

4. Think of throwing that racket over the fence.

5. Concentrate on getting your whole body into the serve.

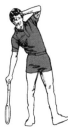

# *Trouble Shooting*—*Serve*

| Trouble | Probable Reason | Try This: |
|---|---|---|
| • serve too long | • leading with wrist<br>• no follow-through, you're pushing the ball | • reach up and snap wrist<br>• reach out into court with body |
| • serve into net | • ball too far in front of you | • toss ball higher<br>• use legs so you hit up into ball |
| • poor ball placement | • poor toss<br>• poor foot placement<br>• incorrect grip | • toss ball farther in front<br>• open your stance<br>• relax hand during backswing |

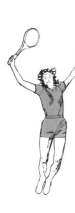

## *Fitness Goals—Serve*

1. *Push* with your legs.
2. *Stretch* your entire right side, from shoulder to hips—up through the ball.
3. *Throw* your right side up and over the ball.
4. *Propel* your right side into the court after the hit. The farther the better. □

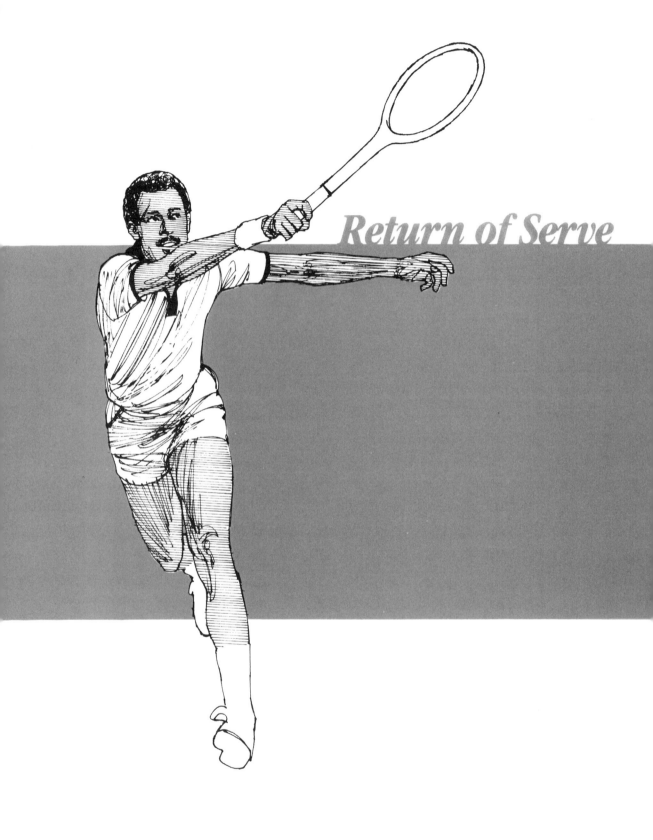

*Return of Serve*

*"Oh no*, here comes that serve." You're often tense because the ball is coming at you harder than a groundstroke. You're nervous because you're thinking you must clobber it back. So you freeze up and don't move well to get the incoming serve.

Don't worry about smoking it back. Block it, chip it, chop it. Just *concentrate on making your opponent hit another ball after the serve.* This will ease your tension. It will help dispel any nervousness about either the serve coming to you, or the thought of knocking it back past your opponent. Your philosophy is to have a *consistent* return and make the server *do* something.

On a return of serve, your stroking action is like that of an abbreviated groundstroke—shorter and more compact. Your frame of mind is like that for a volley—aggressive and positive. If you think, "Hey, all I need to do is block that ball," you'll be amazed at the pace of your return. The server is providing the power for your return. But if you think you have to clobber it, you'll often overswing.

## *Where Do I Stand?*

It will depend on the strength of your opponent's serve. If your opponent has a weak serve, you'll obviously move in closer. If it's a more aggressive serve and bounces deeper, you'll have to stand back.

*Constant Motion... You should always be moving. It's like driving a car. When you glance down at the wheel even when you're on a fairly straight road, your hands are always moving, making slight adjustments. In the same way, when you're playing tennis alertly, you're never standing stock still.*

## *Tune In Early*

Do you sometimes stand there petrified—and then all of a sudden the ball comes roaring in? Just tune in to the serve. Focus on the ball the minute it's in your opponent's hand. Don't wait until it's tossed in the air. Keep your eyes riveted on the ball. Watch the *whole action.* This gets you into the swing of things—gears you up.

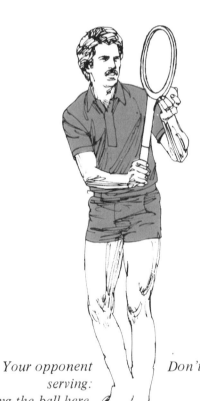

*Your opponent serving: Start watching the ball here.*

*Don't wait to start watching until the ball is here.*

It not only prepares you to react early, but, again, it gives you something to concentrate on and quiets your mind. Don't just be reacting to the ball coming at you.

In the 1982 Wimbledon championships, Jimmy Connors was asked how he handled John Alexander's tough serve. He said the key was to tune in early and watch the ball from the time it was tossed. From this he got into the swing of the return and was able to pick out—very early—the spot Alexander was going to serve to.

## Clues for Overcoming Anxiety

If you are anxious, you're too worried about what *you're* going to do. You're overthinking. Block out those thoughts and try to pick out the *clues* your opponent is giving you as to where he or she is going to serve the ball:

- If the ball is thrown back over the server's head, it must have spin to go in. It will have some hop and will always bounce to the left. But it will be difficult for the server to hit it wide.
- If it's thrown over to the right, it's going to have a slice. It will bounce to your right and stay low. Watch out for this serve in the forehand court.
- If the toss is very high, it's probably going to be very hard and flat, and you'll have to stay back a bit.
- If the toss is low, it's probably going to be flat lollipop—easy to hit. Get ready to move in.
- If the server stands close to the center marker, you are vulnerable down the middle of the court. The wider he stands the wider you will be drawn.

It's helpful to remember you don't have to break serve every time. My college coach always reminded us that to win a match we only had to break serve once per set (assuming of course we were serving well). This took a lot of pressure off.

## Go Meet It

Imagine that you are standing in a doorway, waiting for that serve. There's a chair just behind you.

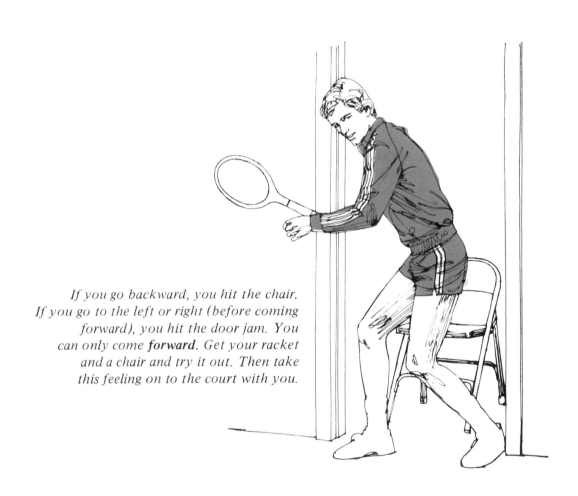

*If you go backward, you hit the chair. If you go to the left or right (before coming forward), you hit the door jam. You can only come **forward**. Get your racket and a chair and try it out. Then take this feeling on to the court with you.*

## *Move Early*

Once you've trained yourself to move only *forward,* keep thinking of the word *early.* Move into the ball early and your weight will be behind the shot. Don't take your racket back behind your body. Keep the racket behind the ball.

If your opponent has a high bouncing serve, taking it early will stop it from bouncing over your head. If you take a slice early, you'll be hitting it before it travels any further away from you.

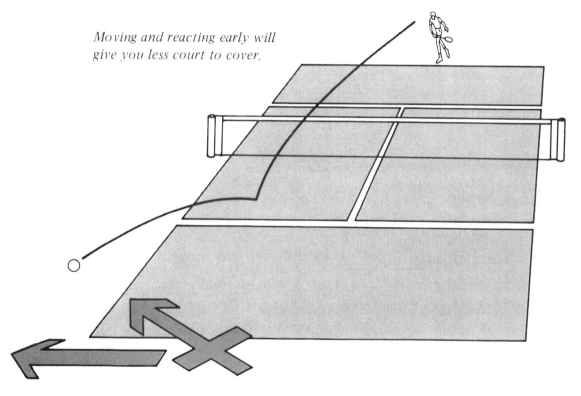

*Moving and reacting early will give you less court to cover.*

Because a good server can have the ball coming at you in so many different ways, you'll have to be flexible and hit the ball from many positions.

## *First Game: Hit Out*

When you start a match, you're often nervous. You'll just push the ball around. To loosen up in the first game, try being more aggressive. "I may lose this first game but, doggone it, I'm going to move!" Hit through the ball.

## *Don't Just Bounce—Pounce!*

How many times has someone told you, "Bounce—get on your toes," in preparing for a return? Certainly you want your legs to feel alive.

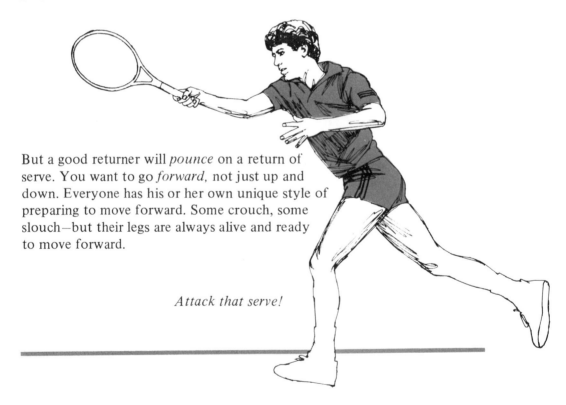

But a good returner will *pounce* on a return of serve. You want to go *forward,* not just up and down. Everyone has his or her own unique style of preparing to move forward. Some crouch, some slouch—but their legs are always alive and ready to move forward.

*Attack that serve!*

## *Jimmy the Pouncer*

Years ago, when I lived in Los Angeles, my friend Allen Fox (now the coach at Pepperdine) was describing a 16 year old player who had just moved to L.A. from Illinois. Allen describing his return of serve as ". . . really rough to handle—he just pounces on those serves." The next week, this unknown teenager—Jimmy Connors—beat Roy Emerson, then one of the world's best players, and his career was on its way—characterized then as now by a tremendously aggressive and consistent return of serve.

## *You Don't Have to Stay Back*

If you go forward to pounce on the ball, you will find yourself closer to the net than usual. Why retreat? Keep going. Become more offensive. Don't worry about where you hit the shot from. You may end up in no-man's land, but you may also hit a great return.

## *Don't Step Sideways*

Concentrate on using your whole body. It will help you in your return of serve more than any other shot. Wherever that ball is hit to you on the serve, you have to get your body behind it. If you don't, there won't be any zip in your return. This summer in Vail I was working on returns of serve with a class. I was serving and they were returning. Most of the players would get their racket behind the ball—they were ready—then they'd take that horrible step sideways. They were prepared; but then, by thinking "sideways to the net . . .," they became unprepared. They couldn't stand to have it simple. Remember: Turn your shoulders, get your racket back and move forward—and your body will be behind the shot.

## Pick a Target

Do you have a target or are you just pushing the ball back? What helps me in returning serves well is to do some positive thinking, to have a visual image. I think of looking down a culvert or a tunnel. I picture where I want the ball to go.

## Your Own Style

Pick out the things you do well on groundstrokes and volleys and incorporate them into your returns of serve. If your groundstrokes are powerful, use them aggressively on returns of serve. If you enjoy quickness at the net, capitalize on that strength by stepping into the return, taking the ball early and coming into the net behind it when you can.

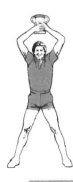

## Tips—Return of Serve

There are two key words to remember:

- Forward
- Early

You must always move forward and you must react early.

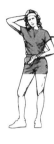

# *Trouble Shooting—Return of Serve*

| Trouble | Probable Reason | Try This |
|---------|-----------------|----------|
| ● return too long | ● you're nervous and not stepping into ball and following through | ● point racket at target at end of hit <br><br> awaken your legs |
| ● return too short or into net | ● no lift | ● bend knees and stay down |
| ● poor ball placement | ● ball taken too late | ● pick a target <br> ● prepare early and meet ball early |

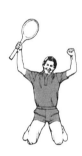

# *Fitness Goals—Return of Serve*

1. *Get low* and work your legs.
2. *Guide* the ball. Don't let it guide you.
3. *Run* back to the baseline or sprint forward. Move after the hit. □

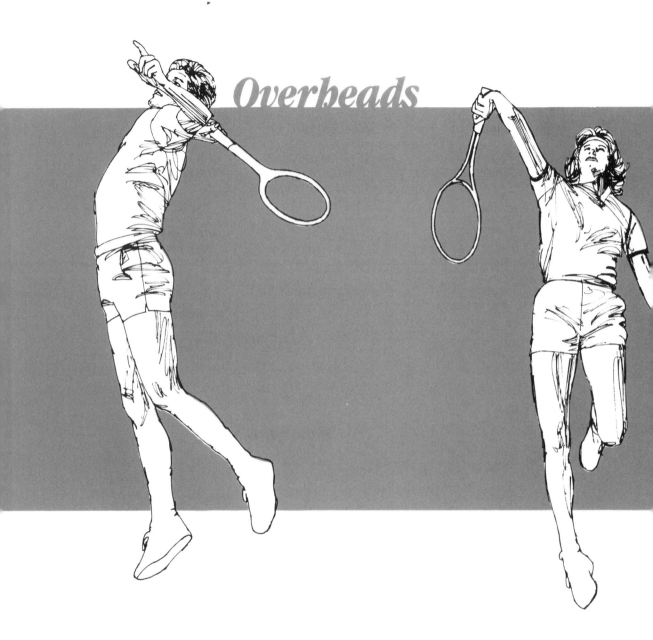

*Overheads*

*The overhead* is like a serve with legs. In a serve you're confined behind the baseline; with an overhead you can (and must) move your legs and run to get under the ball.

The overhead is also a serve without the toss. The ball is placed there for you. This makes it simpler, and you don't have to worry about both a hit *and* a toss.

Even though the overhead is similar to a serve, it doesn't follow that a good server automatically has a good overhead or vice-versa. There are many players—both men and women—who have an average serve and a devastating overhead. For example, Ken Rosewall never had an over-powering serve, yet his overhead was deadly. He was the perfect picture of a player who followed the requirements of hitting good overheads. These are the qualities you need:

- *Quickness:* You move your feet quickly and get behind the ball.
- *Assertiveness:* You reach up and go for the ball.

Remember it's a *smash*—not a push or a poke. You must be positive and spontaneous.

## Don't Get Caught Flat-Footed

Look for these clues: your opponent is:

- Leaning back.
- Opening the racket face.
- Starting an abbreviated swing.

When you see any of this happening, you can start backpedaling because you can bet your boots it's going to be a lob.

## Where Should I Start?

When you anticipate or see a lob coming at you, move back. Of course, if you are an exceptionally good athlete you can play very close to the net. In college, my doubles partner could jump through the ceiling and he'd play with his nose hanging over the net. Throughout four years of playing with him, I can hardly ever remember a ball getting over his head—he'd just jump up and smash every one.

## Don't Be a Statue

Watching a high overhead drift down into the court can be mesmerizing. Don't just stand still. Keep your feet moving. Many good players keep their rackets moving while waiting for an overhead. It helps them relax and stay flexible.

## Why Do You Miss Easy Overheads?

Because, finally, you've set up the point—you're in a position to win it, and this makes you over-anxious. You don't watch the ball, you look at the spot you want it to go. "But that ball was just sitting up there. How could I miss it?" This happens to experienced players as well as beginners. One player recently said to me, "There's something about an overhead that demagnetizes my racket."

## Pointing Is Polite Here

Everyone says, "Use your left hand—point at the ball." It doesn't do any good to point at the ball unless you *watch* the ball all the way through. So *do* point your left hand at the ball, but keep your eye fastened on it and swing through the ball to the spot where you want it to go.

*Point at the ball, turn your shoulders.*

## *Hit In Front*

You already have the advantage of hitting down on the ball. We are often taught to hit the ball at the highest point we can. You *do* want to hit the ball high, but it's just as important to get the ball in front of you so you get your body moving forward.

## *You Don't Have to Be Wilt the Stilt*

The overhead smash is like a spike in volleyball or a slam-dunk in basketball. But in both those sports you have to be relatively tall to execute such plays. In tennis you do not—the net is only 36" high. When you do hit a good overhead, it's a real feeling of power. You feel like a star. You make a tremendous push/leap/propulsion up into the ball, and then hit it down. There is an exuberance and thrill in hitting it well.

## *Go for It!*

This is the shot you've been looking for. Your opponent has probably hit you a lob from a defensive position, is in trouble and vulnerable. Don't let him off the hook by being indecisive. Pick a spot and go for it. The idea isn't to keep the ball in play, but to put it away. Use a throwing action with your full body behind it.

## *Don't Relax*

After hitting the overhead, don't count your opponent out and let your guard down. Be ready—physically and psychologically—to hit another shot. Anticipate that he may run it down and hit it back. Also, if you concentrate on preparing for another hit after your smash, you'll be amazed at how your follow-through will improve.

## *Chance for a Workout*

We've all phantasized that we have performed some heroic athletic feat. Catching a TD pass, beating Tracy Austin . . . here's your chance to be a running jumping athlete. There is nothing more exciting in tennis than backpedaling quickly for a ball overhead, then leaping and smashing it for a winner. Here you have the spike, a slam-dunk and home run all rolled into one.

### *Turn Off Your Mind*

Even though you may concentrate intensely on analyzing your strokes in practice, try to limit your conscious thinking while playing. In no other stroke is this more vital than in the overhead. The more you think about it, the worse the shot is going to be. The fluidity of the shot is lost. When you over-analyze it, you don't put any body behind it and your stroke is short and pokey.

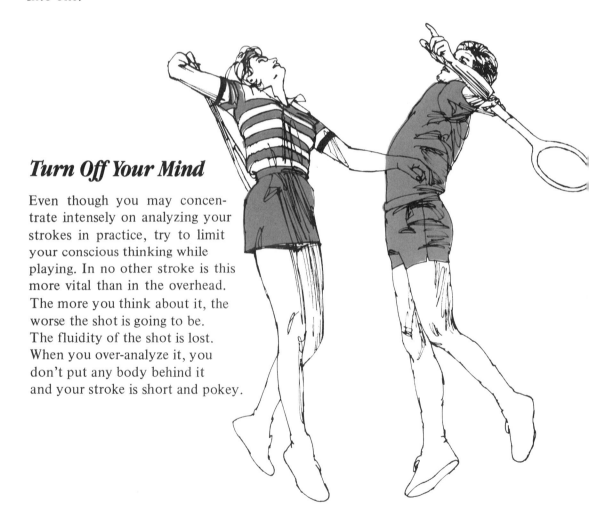

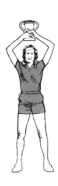

# *Tips—Overheads*

1. Reach with your left hand toward the ball. It lines up the ball and your shoulder.
2. Feel the use of your upper body muscles.
3. Recover after the hit and *bounce back* to an offensive position at the net.
4. Guide your racket through the ball.

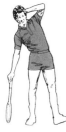

# *Trouble Shooting—Overheads*

| Trouble | Probable Reason | Try This |
|---------|-----------------|----------|
| ● smash too long | ● too lazy or slow and ball gets behind you | ● hit in front of you |
| ● smash too short—into net | ● ducking your head, not watching the ball | ● keep shoulders, arm, chest open and up, hitting up into ball |

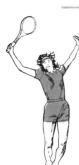

# *Fitness Goals—Overheads*

1. *Sprint* back underneath the ball.
2. *Push* your legs up into the ball.
3. *Propel* your whole hitting side up and through the ball. □

# Lobs and Half-Volleys

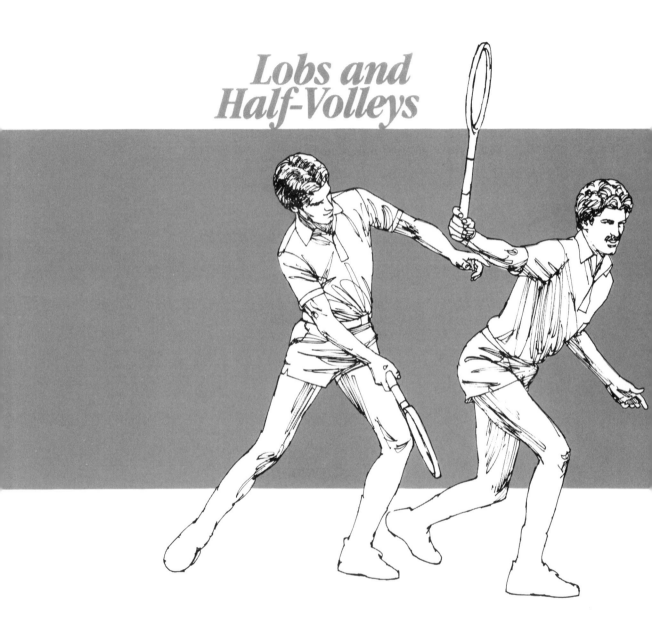

*What a weapon!* Don't apologize for using it. The lob is one of the most useful tools in your bag of tricks.

First, the lob is not a sign of weakness. It has many purposes. It may be an admission of your poor court position, but it is also a sign of intelligence, adaptability and fight—your desire to stay in the point.

## It Ain't What It Used to Be

One of the great pastimes of sports fans is the endless debate over, "Who's better?" among players of a different era. Would Martina Navratilova have beat Althea Gibson or Helen Wills? Would Lendl or McEnroe have beat Don Budge, Jack Kramer or Ellsworth Vines? These questions are never resolved. However, in the arsenal of every world class tennis player today is a weapon that has been perfected way beyond what it was in the "old" days: the topspin lob. Those dazzling topspin lobs, as hit by Andrea Jaeger or John McEnroe (with tremendously exaggerated low-to-high swing), are the only way to get the ball over the head of an agile, aggressive volleyer.

## A Variable Weapon

Think for a minute what the lob does and you'll wonder why it is given such cursory treatment in most tennis books. It can:

- Give you time to get back into position during a baseline rally.
- Pry that aggressive net rusher away from the net.
- Be hit with disguise and topspin for outright winners.
- Be used tactically as a change of pace to break up the rhythm of a ground-stroking opponent.

# *Threat of a Lob*

When your opponent comes to the net, you can do one of three things:
Hit to the right, hit to the left or lob over his head. If he knows you won't
lob, he'll come in close to the net where he can reach your passing shots.
But if he knows you might lob, he has to stay back; this gives you more
room to hit those passing shots to the right or left.

# *Lay It on a Cloud*

Think of a big cloud in the sky above the courts. Lay the ball on that
cloud. Don't hit it, place it there. Slow the ball down and hit it
softly, delicately. If you've played golf, think of your last chip
shot from 50 yards which landed softly on the green. Your
approach to the lob is the same: Lift the ball into the air gently,
with feeling, by opening your racket face.

*Lower to higher;
more bend, more lift*

## Lob Up the Ski Lift

Make your racket go up a steeper ski lift; start lower and end higher than on a normal groundstroke.

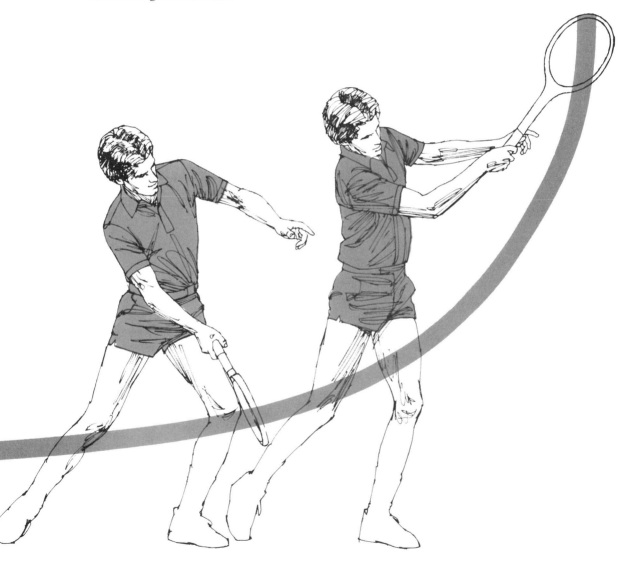

## Open Your Racket Face

Picture a high fence 3 to 4 feet on the other side of the net and open up your racket face to hit the lob over that imaginary obstacle. This keeps your attention focused on the ball and target, and keeps your opponent out of your field of concentration.

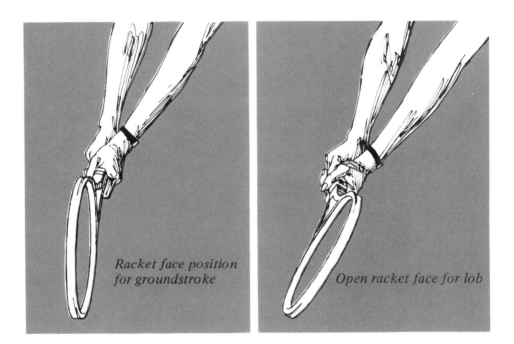

*Racket face position for groundstroke*

*Open racket face for lob*

## Disguise Helps

If you open your racket face prior to the hit, or lean back, your opponent will know you're going to lob. A good way to disguise a lob is to bend your knees, drop your shoulder, lower the racket head and come up on the ball from below it—just like you do on a groundstroke.

## Move Forward

Keep moving forward. As in groundstrokes, keep the legs and body working—to get a better workout, and to be a more effective player. This will give you a more positive lob and help disguise the shot. You can even exaggerate—really step in, move forward—but throw up the lob at the last minute.

## Focus on the Ball

Bill Tilden used to say that watching a ball is like depth of field in focusing a camera. You can either have the ball clear and the background fuzzy, or vice-versa. On a lob, there is an almost irresistible tendency to take a peek at your opponent. Resist this, and keep the ball in focus. Peripheral view of your opponent is good enough.

## Spin

For a defensive lob, you want a little underspin on the ball—just like on a low volley—to give you control and lift. A quarterback wouldn't expect to hit the target if he threw the ball end-over-end. It has to spin. If you hit with underspin, you can hit the ball softly.

## After You Lob

You're going to have to run. If your lob is weak, you'll have to run down another overhead. If you have to go on the defensive, have fun defending, running and blocking the ball back deep. If you hit a good lob over your opponent's head, you'll usually want to run up to take the net away from your opponent. So whatever happens, get on your running shoes. That's what you're out there for.

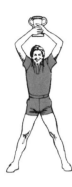

# *Tips—Lobs*

1. Forget about form with a lob. Do anything to get the ball back up there.
2. If you have to miss a lob, err on the side of hitting it long. This will help you hit through the ball.
3. Disguise it as long as you can. The longer you keep your opponent at the net, the easier it is to lob over her head.

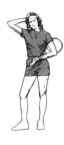

# *Trouble Shooting—Lobs*

| Trouble | Probable Reason | Try This |
|---|---|---|
| ● lob over the baseline | ● overhitting <br> ● too big a swing | ● shorten swing <br> ● keep ball on strings |
| ● lob too short | ● looking up too soon | ● aim for baseline |

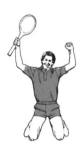

# *Fitness Goals—Lobs*

1. Use legs and body to *lift* ball up over opponent's head.
2. After your lob, recover and be ready to *run* or *dive* in the opposite direction. □

# *Half-Volleys*

The poor half-volley—it's tennis' stepchild; and the way it's usually taught, it's no wonder we miss so many. We're warned about never getting caught in the dreaded "no man's land": the area of the court between the service line and three to four feet inside the baseline.

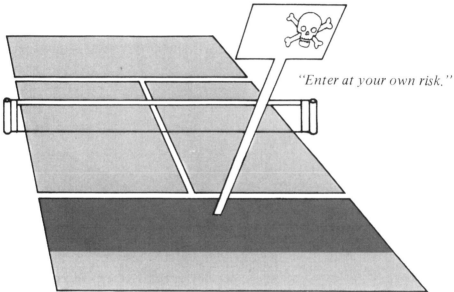

*"Enter at your own risk."*

When we *are* caught there, our usual response is, "I'll hit the ball here 'real quick' and get to the net where I should be—maybe no one will see me." This thinking causes a lot of troubled half-volleys.

You're going to have to hit some half-volleys in every match. Remember, even the quickest player is going to get caught mid-court. Don't rush through mid-court to get to a volleying position at the net just because you're afraid of being caught in no-man's land. This greatly hinders your ability to move laterally. Remember you have to *stop*—regardless of your court position—when your opponent hits the ball. Give the half-volley a chance and it can be an enjoyable, effective shot. Let's find out what it is, then use it to help us play better.

## *What Is It Anyway?*

A "half-volley"? If it hits the ground, how can it be a volley, even half of one? It's like a volley in that it's hit close to the net with a very short back swing. But that's as close to a volley as it gets. It's actually a short compact groundstroke, hit very soon after it bounces. Try thinking of it as *half* a groundstroke taken *half* way to the net.

You're forced into this shot because *you want to be moving forward.* It's similar to fielding a grounder in baseball. If you don't take it early after the hop it will bounce over your head.

## *It's Part Groundstroke*

It's hit close to the net, but the rest of the shot is pure groundstroke:

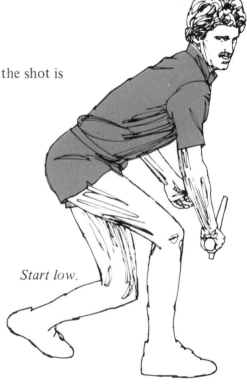

- Bend early and deeply.
- Swing low to high.
- Take the ball in front.

*Start low.*

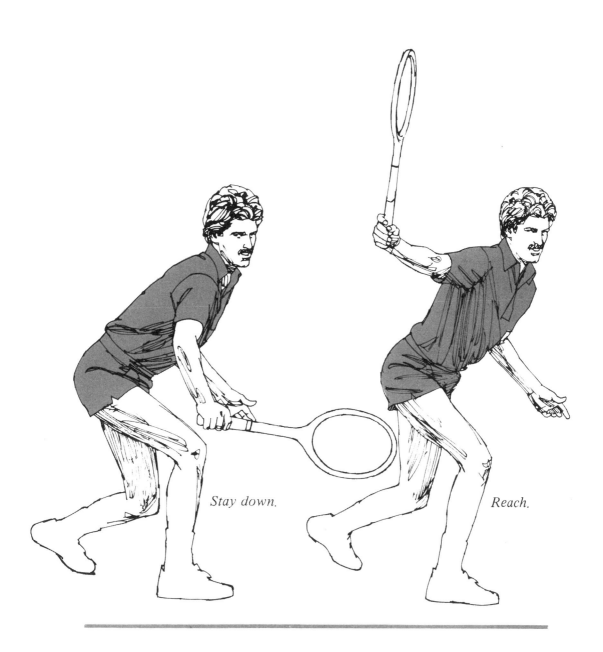

*Stay down.*

*Reach.*

## *Low Down*

You're fairly limited in what you can do with the half-volley. Face it. When you have to hit this shot you're on the defensive. The best you can do is hit the ball deep along the baseline to keep your opponent back, or low over the net if he has taken a net position. The key to doing this is to stay low and down with the ball.

## *Work on It and Get a Workout*

Hitting a half-volley deeply and crisply is one of the most enjoyable experiences in tennis. You get down to the ball and hit it in front of you. You use your feet to get behind the ball and your body to hit through it. Next time you practice, spend 10 minutes taking only half-volleys. Then if you continue the drill—working farther back—you'll soon find yourself on the baseline, taking your groundstrokes earlier and earlier, and improving them. You'll get a terrific workout, your conditioning will improve and your reactions to every ball will be speeded up.

## *Enjoy the Trip*

As your half-volleys improve, you will find your net game improving also. Instead of flying through the middle of the court—or no man's land—relax when you are caught there. When you're more relaxed, your lateral movement will be better. Your view of your net game will change and you will enjoy the trip to the net.

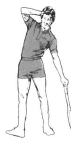

# *Trouble Shooting—* **Half-Volleys**

| Trouble | Probable Reason | Try This |
|---------|-----------------|----------|
| ● half-volley too long | ● you stood up too soon | ● bend knees and stay down<br>● hit ball in front |
| ● ball too short or into net | ● didn't get below ball | ● stop as soon as opponent hits & get down |

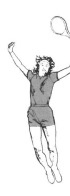

# *Fitness Goals—* **Half-Volleys**

1. *Bend* with your legs, not your back.
2. *Push* forward, take ball early—don't sit back.
3. *Fight* urge to pull up. Stay down and reach forward. □

**Use Your Whole Body** . . . *I'm not saying, "Don't use your wrist," but rather, "Back up your wrist with your whole body." Dancers have always been aware of total body involvement. Now other athletes are catching on to the importance of using the whole rather than parts of the body.*

# *Spin*

*"But the pro at my club* told me to hit every ball with topspin," a student told me recently. I explained that not every ball that's hit to her *can* be hit with topspin, and further, that there are other types of spin that may be more suitable for her natural playing style.

In the chapter on groundstrokes, we talked about using and improving on your own style and not slavishly copying anyone else's. The same applies to spin. There's not one spin that everyone should use; every player uses a different combination of spins. The same player that just hit an underspin backhand approach shot may have to hit over the ball with topspin to pass an opponent at the net on the very next point. The ability to vary spin is the mark of a top player. Not every great shot has the same kind of spin. Rosewall has an underspin backhand. Segura has a little top-spin on his great forehand; both Chris Evert-Lloyd and Tracy Austin have a little spin on their back-hands, but some spin on their forehands; Bjorn Borg's forehand has a lot of topspin; Martina Navratilova has a lot of topspin on her forehand and underspin on her backhand.

*Underspin: high to low*

## *Types of Spin*

There's nothing mysterious about spin. Every ball has it—that TD pass, that curve over the corner of the plate, that service ace.

*Underspin* makes the ball rise. It's a control mechanism. It takes some speed off the ball but gives you control. Every low volley should be hit with some underspin; you can also use it on some groundstrokes, drop shots and some lobs. To get underspin start with your racket above the ball and hit slightly down and through it, toward the target. Go from shoulder height to your waist, with a pulling-down action. Underspin is somewhat limited because the harder you hit the ball the more it sails. Rosewall gets away with it because he hits right *through* the ball.

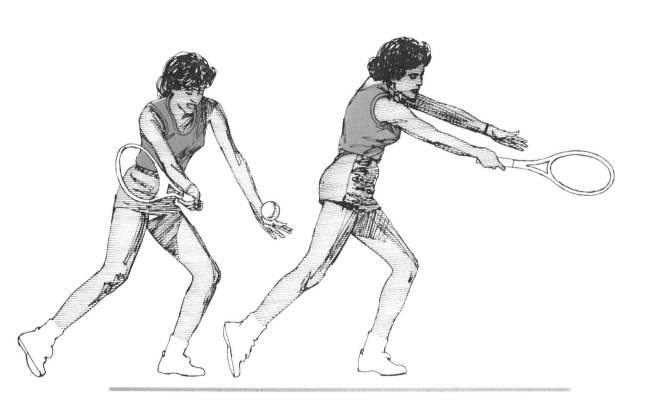

*Topspin* makes the ball drop. It's the most common type of spin, and the most effective for beginners. People often describe it as "brushing over" the ball. But this causes problems. To get topspin, think: Hit *through* the ball from a point that's low to a point that's high. Go from your knee to your shoulder.

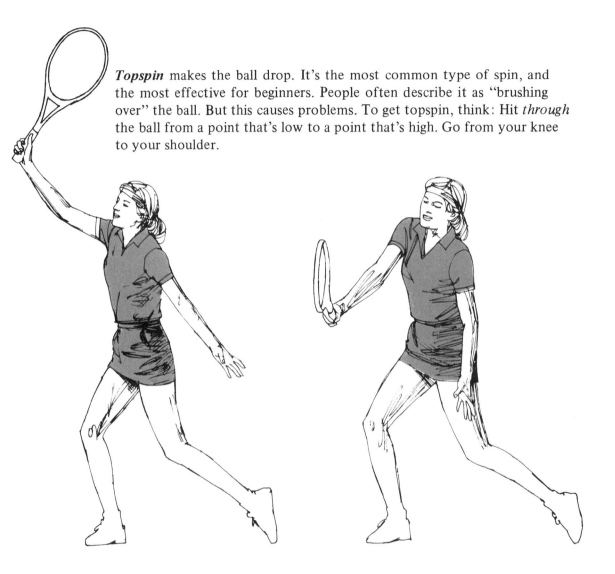

*Sidespin:* You come across from outside the ball to inside the ball with a brushing action. Just slide the ball to the desired spot. Sidespin is used mostly for approach shots and balls below the net level.

## *Your Own Particular Spin*

Don't copy someone else's spin. It will set you back. Many young players tried to copy Borg's topspin after watching him play, with less-than-satisfactory results. What spin you'll use should depend upon whatever gives you the most control and whatever feels most natural.

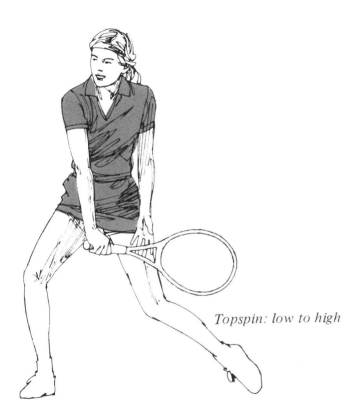

*Topspin: low to high*

Practice the different spins in drills or rallies. See which suits you best. Then when you're playing a match, don't be mechanical—stay flexible. There won't be one spin for every shot.

***The Myth of the Natural Athlete*** . . . *Some people obviously have more natural talent than others, but all of us can play good tennis. For example, Bruce Jenner was a mediocre athlete in high school and through hard work (6 to 8 hours a day for four years), became a gold-medal decathlon winner. Tai Babilonia, the Olympic skating star and 1979 World Pair Skating Champion, says she wasn't a natural athlete. She couldn't skate at all when she first tried it but practiced for three hours before school and four hours after school every day. You won't be going to these extremes, but it **is** reassuring to think that being a good tennis player isn't a "gift" you're born with, but something you can work toward with a good positive attitude.*

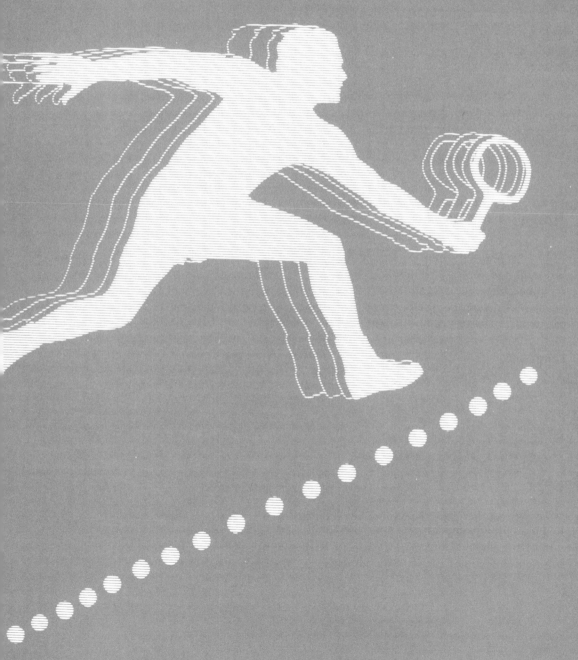

# III. Strategy
# & Tactics

# *Singles*

**When I first began teaching** at a well known tennis ranch, I noticed it didn't take long for beginning students in each clinic to ask the head pro about strategy and tactics. He always answered with a grumble, "When you can learn to hit the damn ball where you want it to go, then we'll talk about strategy." He had a point, but I've found that having an idea of where the ball should go will improve your hitting ability. Learning to hit the ball to a particular spot and knowing the reasons for hitting it there (strategy) go hand in hand with developing your tennis game.

## *Beware of Too Much Strategy*

I've also come to the conclusion that players and coaches who spend a lot of time concocting intricate strategies and match plans are wasting their time. Winning tennis involves simple tactics, executed well. A newspaper report of the McEnroe-Lendl Canadian Open Final of 1982 described a very simple yet winning strategy. Lendl simply got lots of forcing first serves in and if McEnroe *did* hit them back, Lendl overpowered him with his groundstrokes. Lendl simply relied on what he did best. You may not be able to overpower John McEnroe, but you should use the same principles. Keep it simple and do what you do best.

## *Where to Start From*
## *(Not "Where to Stand")*

Remember you are not going to play the entire point from a single spot; it's just a starting place for each particular point. Not every starting position will be the same. Where you start from will vary a great deal depending upon your quickness and the stroking ability of your opponent.

Generally, while playing from the backcourt you should stand 3 to 5 feet behind the baseline. This is a *starting* spot and will probably not be the *hitting* spot. You should try to hit your volleys as close to the net as possible. But be careful not to "camp out" on top of the net. Your position at the net will vary depending upon the quality of your approach shot, your speed, jumping ability and your opponent's ability to lob. These factors will always be changing as will your position at the net. All too often we pick a spot near the net and stay there regardless of changing circumstances.

## *"Hit It Where They Ain't"*

Willie Keeler summed up baseball batting strategy very well when he said, "Hit it where they ain't." We could modify that for our tennis game by saying, "Hit it where it ain't going to come back." Unfortunately, you will seldom be hitting pure aces past your opponent in a match. Most of your points will be won by your opponent's errors, so your strategy is to make him do things he does not do well or does not enjoy doing. That's the best way to generate errors.

## *Be Your Own Scout*

Watch your opponent during the warm-up. Try to discover what he does not do well and try to make him do a lot of that during the match. Don't cut the warm-up short. Take as much time as you need—both to warm up and spot your opponent's weaknesses.

Recently the local sports page had a story on Roger Theder, former head football coach at Cal, who'd just been hired by the Baltimore Colts. His new job was to study the offensive plays of teams the Colts would be playing this season. He was going to analyze what each team did on certain downs in certain parts of the field. We should do the same in tennis. Be aware of what your opponent will generally do in certain positions on the court. You may not have had a chance to see your opponent play a match. But you can make certain game plans just by watching him or her during the warm-up.

## *Where to Hit?*

You will constantly be making judgments about where to hit the ball based on these two things:

- Where do I hit the ball best?
- Where does my opponent hit the ball worst?

Good strategy is a constant combination of these two goals. If you have a wicked cross-court forehand, it would be foolish not to use it. In club tennis, your opponent will generally have a weak backhand; if so, direct the ball to that weak spot as often as possible. And you'll want to carefully test your opponent's overhead. It may be weak and make his net attack more vulnerable.

If your opponent's backhand and forehand are roughly equal in strength, most of your groundstrokes should go cross-court to take advantage of the lower net (in the middle), increased court area and your better position after hitting the ball cross-court. There will almost always be a weaker side (forehand or backhand) to hit to, as this opponent with equal forehand and backhand strengths probably does not exist.

## *There Are No Bad Spots*

But some are better than others. Do you know why? Because of the constant movement of tennis you'll have to hit the ball from many different spots. The earlier you are aware of this in your tennis career the better. Too often we get limited by thinking we can only hit a good shot from a particular spot. You may have to hit a half-volley from a yard inside the baseline. Or you may hit a winning passing shot with your back up against the fence. There are no batter's boxes in tennis. You can hit any shot from any location.

Some very important matches have been won by players who maintained their sense of imagination and experimented with returning serves from way inside the baseline, or by standing several yards behind the baseline. The late Raphael Osuna won the U.S. Open in 1964 by returning Frank Froehling's huge serve from 12 to 15 feet behind the baseline. Be flexible. Start from a spot that feels natural and evaluate the results.

## Comfort Isn't Everything

One of my team players will often say something to me like, "Well coach, I feel comfortable standing inside the baseline while returning a serve." And I'll say, "You may be comfortable there but you haven't hit a ball in the court in the last two sets." You must constantly evaluate results.

Some of the most effective serves in women's club tennis are those that barely sneak over the net. They work because the receiving player feels she must wait for these serves behind the baseline. These serves will lose their effectiveness when the receiver realizes she may have to move in much closer than she normally would.

While no man's land isn't necessarily where you *want* to hit from, you must acknowledge that you are going to have to hit some balls there—either on your way to the net with a volley or while retreating from the net with an overhead. Don't worry if you are caught in no man's land. You can hit great shots from there and not receive the death sentence for failure to get to the net more quickly.

## Changing Tactics

Larry Stefanki, an outstanding player on our Cal team in 1979, was playing an important match against San Jose State. We had spent a lot of time trying to improve Larry's groundstrokes. During this match against a player who was a good groundstroker, Larry stayed in the backcourt—as he had been doing during practice. This would have been fine if he'd wanted to practice his groundstrokes, but he was behind and we needed to win this match. I remember going down to him at the end of the first set: "Larry, you're playing very well from the backcourt, but this guy is good in the backcourt too. Get to the net where you are at your best." So he started coming into the net and won the match easily after that. He was practicing his groundstrokes, but he wasn't winning. He changed to a strategy that was a stronger part of his game.

## *Try Something New*

In the 1982 Northern California Intercollegiate Championships, our number one player at Cal, Randy Nixon, was to play Stanford's top player, Scott Davis. Scott had beaten Randy earlier that year and on many occasions before that. I told Randy before the match, "You've got nothing to lose, so try something different." Randy went out and forced the play every chance he got. He served and came into the net behind every ball, and on every short serve would hit the ball and come into the net. He was more aggressive and took more chances than he normally would and went on to win the match.

Especially if you're losing a big match, try something new. Experiment. Loosen up: "I've got nothing to lose." You can never overestimate the value of surprise. Serve and come to the net when you have been staying in the back court; chip a short serve return and come to the net behind it; hit a semi-lob and sneak into the net behind it.

These may be simple tactics that will turn the match around. They will also make the match more of an adventure. Only *you* keep yourself stuck in that rut. *You* can make the decision to do something different. Try it. Your game may never be the same again.

## *Post-Match Review*

A grizzly old law school professor of mine at Denver University used to lecture us immediately after we had taken an exam—that *now*, since everything was fresh in our minds—was the time to study. We, of course, thought he was crazy, but now I understand he was right.

It's very difficult to analyze a match immediately after it is completed. If you win, you want to celebrate; if you lose, you want to forget it as soon as possible. There is something to be said for both approaches. You do not want to lose any of the excitement or enthusiasm of a hard fought victory, nor do you want to dwell forever upon a loss. But let's try the middle course.

If you win, analyze what you've done correctly, put that on a recorder in your mind, remember that method and try to recreate those winning plays and shots. Use them again.

I tell my Cal team: If you lose, analyze what you did well, what you did not do so well, and face squarely what you did not do well at all. This will be the basis for hard work and improvement. Only by recognizing your weaknesses and working on them can you improve.

In the 1978 U.S.-Mexican Davis Cup tie in Tucson, U.S. Captain Tony Trabert rushed over to Roscoe Tanner after Tanner's key win over Raul Ramariz, not simply to congratulate him, but to re-emphasize some of the reasons that he won the match. Trabert and Tanner were already thinking about the next match.

*You're Always at Bat . . . John Gaynor, a friend of mine in Reno, Nevada and a former college football player, recently said to me, "I wish I'd started playing tennis when I was 12 or 13." He said it was impossible to go out and find 10 other guys to play football with, whereas in tennis all he needed was one. Other advantages of tennis, as compared to team sports, are that the ball is hit to you every time, you have control of the tempo and you never get taken out of the game after a bad shot. You're the pitcher, catcher and hitter all in one.*

# Questions Everybody Asks About Doubles

Playing doubles is one of the most exciting events in sports. Having a partner standing next to you can do much to ease the seriousness and sometime grimness of a singles match. Your partner will share the joy of the good shots and winning matches and help ease the pain of tough losses. Here tennis becomes a team game. These are some of the most commonly asked questions about playing doubles:

*Who Should I Pick for My Partner?* Your best partner may not be the best singles player in the club. You are looking for someone who will compliment your game. If you're a big hitter, you'll want to find a partner who is very steady but maybe not sensational. If you are the steady one, you may be looking for someone with a lot of power to take advantage of all the balls you get back in the court.

*Should I Always Come to the Net?* If you're very athletic and have a good overhead, by all means, live at the net. But if you're not that comfortable up there, pick your approaches to the net discreetly. Only come in when your opponent's shot is very short and has already drawn you in toward the net.

*Must We both Move Together at All Times?* Must you always play side by side? Ideally, this is terrific. But most of your doubles play will be with one up and one back, which is o.k. as long as the net person does not become a mere spectator.

*Who Cover Overheads?* Try to take all balls over your head. Run, leap, extend yourself—this is what you're out there for. No more ducking your head, shouting, "Yours!" and scurrying to the other side of the court.

*When Should I Lob?* You *must* lob when your opponents are dug in at the net. You *may* lob when you're pinned deep along the baseline, when you need time to get back into the court or when your opponent has hit a very "big" shot.

***When Can I Poach?*** You can poach any time you want. Just don't miss, kid.

***Who Covers the Ball Hit Up the Middle?*** The one with the strong forehand.

***Where Do I Go when My Partner is Drawn Wide?*** You must cover the middle.

***When I'm at the Net, When Do I Cover the Middle?*** When your opponents are returning from the middle of the court. (See below.)

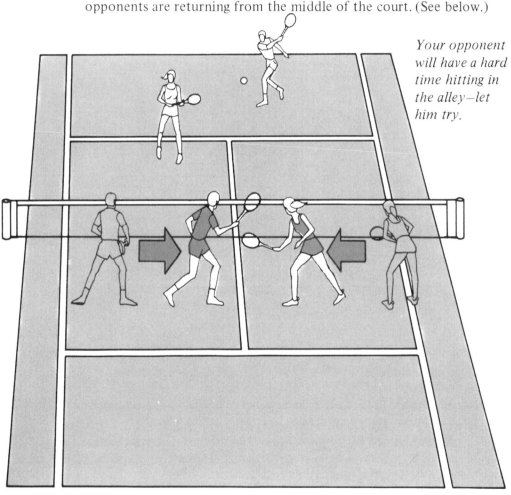

*Your opponent will have a hard time hitting in the alley—let him try.*

**When I'm At the Net, When Do I Cover the Alley?** Whenever your opponent hits the ball from the sidelines (See below.)

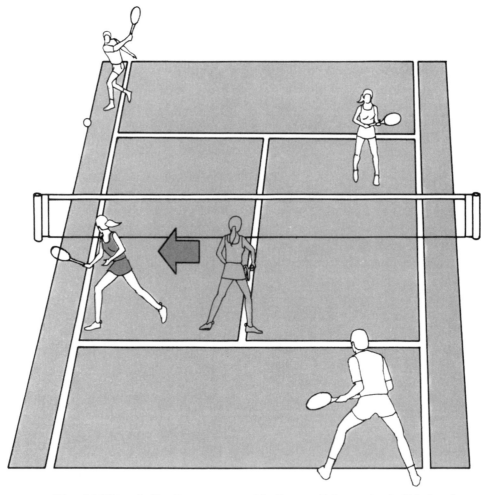

**Should I Watch My Opponent or My Partner?** Once the ball is in play always watch your partner hit the ball. This will give you an added jump in reaction time.

***Where Should I Stand when My Partner Returns A Serve?*** Start in a position where you can cover your partner's typical return.

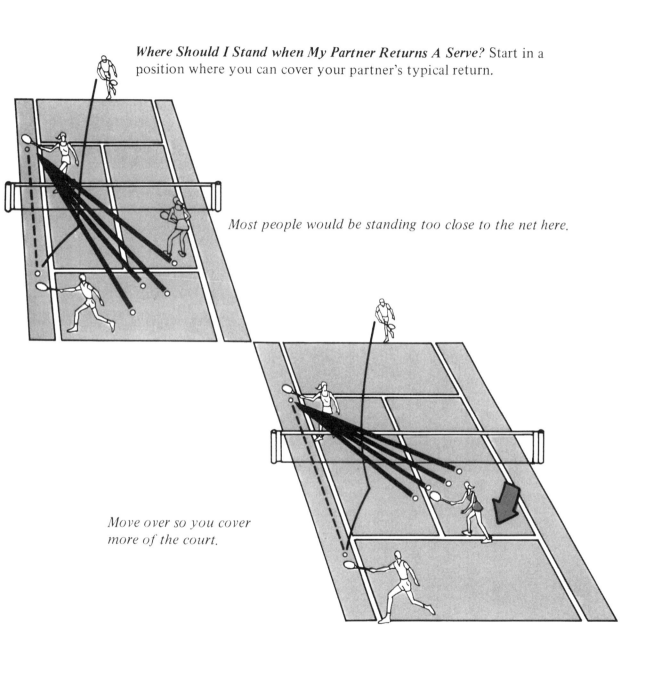

*Most people would be standing too close to the net here.*

*Move over so you cover more of the court.*

***Where Do I Go when My Partner Hits a Good Cross-Court Return?***
Closer to the net and in a position to poach.

***Should We Talk?*** Certainly. You must communicate. For example, when the ball bounces down the middle and could be hit by either of you, the player with the strongest shot should call for it. □

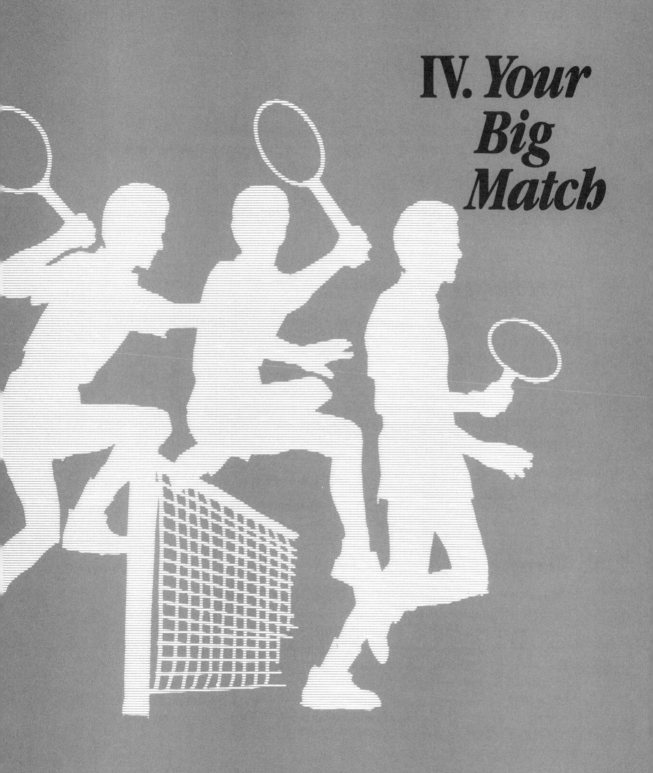

# IV. Your Big Match

**The Wimbledon finals** or the Davis Cup are not the only big matches in tennis today. We all have our own big match, the one that really means something to us, where we want to play as well as we can. It may be a match against your business competitor, your boss, or it may be a mixed doubles match where you want your partner to be proud of you. It's a big match if it's important to you.

## Nervous? It's Natural

You will know when your big match is coming. You'll probably be nervous because you'll want to play well. Athletes, actors, performers of all types have always felt those butterflies. Don't be surprised or paralyzed when you feel them. It means that you are gearing up, mentally and physically, to perform at your best. These butterflies will not necessarily go away with time and experience. An extreme example is basketball great Bill Russell who continued to get sick before every game, even after years of college, Olympic and pro basketball experience. This nervousness is a natural response to wanting to play well. Try to keep the concepts of *Aerobic Tennis* in mind: The more you get your whole body involved in hitting the ball, the quicker you'll lose your nervousness.

## Warming Up

The first time I played at Forest Hills showed me the importance of a good warm-up. My opponent took the six balls we were to use for the match. He first practiced his serve by slicing three out of my reach into the forehand court and then spun the other three out wide to my backhand court. The ball boys hadn't arrived yet and by the time I had retrieved all six balls, our umpire said: "Players ready . . . play!" Fortunately I had hit lots of balls before taking the court for the match. The point here: Don't expect your opponent to give you a meaningful warm-up. Be thoroughly warmed up when you take the court.

## *How to Get Ready*

- *Stretch.* Before your warm-up on the court, get your body ready for action by stretching your muscles (see pp. 126-129).

- *Take Time to Warm Up.* Spend 20 to 30 minutes warming up before playing. There's no way you can walk on the court, casually hit five backhands and five forehands, and expect to play well. Some players will want to warm up in the morning for afternoon matches. Others will prefer (or only have time) to take a complete warm-up as close to match-time as possible. Find out which works best for you. Warmed-up muscles are stronger and injuries are less likely.

- *Take Every Ball Early.* Don't wait for it to bounce twice. Get into good habits for this important day. No sloppiness here!

- *Hit Through the Ball.* Stroke out any nervousness or tension. Don't worry if you're hitting over the baseline. Use this time to get loose and warm.

- *Exaggerate.* When you're hitting the ball, try to get your entire body involved in every shot. Exaggerate bending, reaching and stretching. If you tend to be lazy at the start of a match or are a slow starter, exaggerate everything you do in the warm-up. If you are tentative about coming in to the net, play some points where you come in every time you can in your warm-up.

- *Get Your Blood Circulating.* Serve several games and play out the points. Get in a competitive mood. Try as hard as you can to win these warm-up points. Often we're too casual before the match.

- *Be Positive.* Don't fret about the way you are hitting a particular shot. It's too late to change your stroke.

- *Move!* One sure sign of nervousness is lead feet. Exaggerate move-ment. Run down every ball, even the wide ones, and try to hit them on the first bounce. Then, when the match starts, keep moving. It will help overcome the butterflies.

- *Have a Plan.* It doesn't have to be elaborate, but have a general idea of what you're going to do. You'll be more relaxed if you have a plan of attack, rather than merely responding to your opponent's play. Coach John Wooden's great UCLA basketball teams were a perfect example: They concentrated on their own game plans and didn't spend much time scouting and worrying about what their opponents would do. The plan can be very simple: Pick a spot to serve to, pick a spot to hit groundstrokes to, or work out a pre-set plan to either come to the net or stay back. Formulating these things will give your game (and mind) some direction, and ease your nervousness. Pancho Gonzales used to play the match in his mind prior to taking the court. He pictured himself in a positive manner, serving aggressively, moving to the net, hitting great volleys. Others have pictured themselves handling every situation in a cool, calm, deliberate way.

● *Put the Match in Perspective.* This may be the most important match in your life to date but there will be others. Think of it as a step in your development as a tennis player. Those errors (that are bound to come) won't be so shattering.

● *Your Own Special Preparation.* Just as your own strokes have an individual stamp, so will your preparation. Each of you will find a different recipe for pre-match relaxation. Our Cal team's unorthodox warm-up shocked some coaches at the National Indoor Championships at Princeton in 1980. They caught us using basketball as a pre-game warm-up. We had discovered this technique accidentally one day at a big match when we chanced upon an empty basketball court. " Hey, let's shoot some baskets," said someone. We grabbed a basketball and started to shoot around and soon were in a hotly contested three-on-three game. We played tennis very well that day and have used this unique warm-up as often as we can, much to the amazement of other teams and coaches. It has worked for us, released tension, got us moving and in the mood to compete. (We went on to win the National Indoor Championships that year.)

Some of you will get warmed up listening to music, others by running, still others with rapid-fire volley drills. There isn't one single thing that works for everyone.

## *Enjoy Your Big Match Today*

Maybe you think you'll enjoy playing somewhere down the road when your backhand gets straightened out or your volley is better. These are worthwhile goals, but you'll miss the meaning and fun of tennis if you don't get into today's match with 100% effort and enjoyment. You're out there to have fun and become more fit. Do this and the other goals will take care of themselves.

## *Avoid Labels*

Don't label your opponent or yourself. One of my most consistent mistakes as a coach is to label opponents and their strokes. Without fail the labels are wrong. If I tell one of my Cal players his opponent's backhand is weak, and this opponent has a good day with his backhand, my player will be surprised and discouraged. A better way to approach it would be to say that, generally, this opponent's backhand is not as good as his forehand—but don't be shocked when he hits a backhand winner on a big point.

I learned this the hard way. Years ago, I was eagerly waiting for my match at the Merion Cricket Club with one of the top seeded players, Fred Stolle. Here was my chance for an upset. Stolle hadn't been playing on grass for several weeks. He had done well in the last clay court tournament in Chicago and had only arrived in Philadelphia the night before our match. I thought he would have trouble with the fast grass at Merion and wouldn't be able to adjust, especially to a good serve. When he cracked my first serves back at the start of the match as if he'd been on the grass for the last six months, I was completely shaken. I never recovered and he won easily.

If you label your opponent as "very good" you may be putting her on a pedestal that may make winning impossible. Junior tennis players do this all the time. Or when you label an opponent as "not so good," and she begins to play better than your expectations, you'll be taken by surprise and upset. Try to go into the match with as few preconceived notions as you can. Judge not your opponent, but the balls she's hitting back to you. Remember, you're only playing the ball.

## Use Your Strengths

Forget how someone else thinks you ought to play. You can only enjoy playing when you are relaxed and at ease with your own style. Maybe you are most effective and enjoy playing from the baseline. Then play your big match from there. Don't suddenly become a net rusher because of a match you've just seen on TV. To play well you don't need to play or look like anyone else.

Several years ago, we had a very good player at Cal who was almost unbeatable from the back court, but had trouble when he came to the net. Whenever his teammates finished their matches and watched him play they would tell me, "Coach, tell Scott to get into the net more." I'd say, "Do you know what the score is?" "No." "Well, he's winning." He was more effective and at home on the baseline and this was where he should have been playing his big match.

## Don't Worry About How You Feel

You may get up in the morning and say, "I feel great," and think you'll play great that day. Some of the worst matches have been played by people feeling "great," and some of the best matches have been played by players who have felt lousy. There is no foolproof formula. Keep loose and flexible and go into each match expecting to have to run, jump, stretch and fight. This is the way to prepare.

*Don't Sweat It (Mentally)... You don't have to analyze every miss. Sure, you're going to miss some shots—everyone does. So move on. You're going to make a lot of shots, too.*

# No Sure Formula

Al Attles, coach of the Golden State Warriors, was reminiscing recently about the old days in the National Basketball Association when travel was fairly haphazard. Often his team would struggle all night and get to the gym just minutes before game time—and play tremendously. Other times, travel would be smooth and they'd arrive a day or two ahead of time, and play poorly. You *do* want to prepare well, but sometimes not all the preparation in the world will assure success. The important ingredients to take onto that court with you are your good physical condition and the will to win.

# Don't Pre-judge Yourself

And don't prejudge how you will play. Because you played well yesterday is no guarantee you'll be playing well today. And vice versa. If you've been playing poorly, you now have the chance to step out of your slump and play well. Each day is unique.

# Between Games

In tennis you must be able to go full blast during a point, but you must also know how to let go and relax between points. There was a picture of Arthur Ashe resting during change-over in his 1975 Wimbledon final against Jimmy Connors. Arthur was slumped in a chair with a towel over his head; he looked like he was at the beach. He was calm, relaxed, and conserving energy to prepare for the extreme stress of the next game. It worked—he went on to win.

**The True Meaning of Tennis** . . . *Our games were brutal. No one of us had real put-away shots, nor screaming drives down the sidelines. But we could all place the ball, and it was not unusual for a single point to last two or three minutes before someone was able to smack the ball out of reach.*

*A famous tennis expert came upon us one Sunday morning when the score was 11-12 and deuce in the critical twenty-fourth game. He saw us knocking the ball from side to side, utilizing slices and smashes and lunging recoveries. He covered his face with his hands and said, "This is too painful to watch." He was accustomed to games in which a man served a rocket, ran to the net, and put the ball away. To watch us straining for points through twenty and thirty exchanges, each more cliff-hanging than the preceding, was too enervating.*

*Sometimes, in the excitement of such a game, I would catch the true meaning of tennis: the lovely, shifting figures; the poetic flight of the ball now here, now there; the unexpected drop shot, the arching lob; and always the relation of one player to the other, the figures changing, moving, falling into postures of delicate grace. And I would experience such an overwhelming sense of kinesthesia that when the play finally ended I and the others would cry, "What a great point!" regardless of who had won.*

JAMES A. MICHENER, Sports in America

# V. Stretching

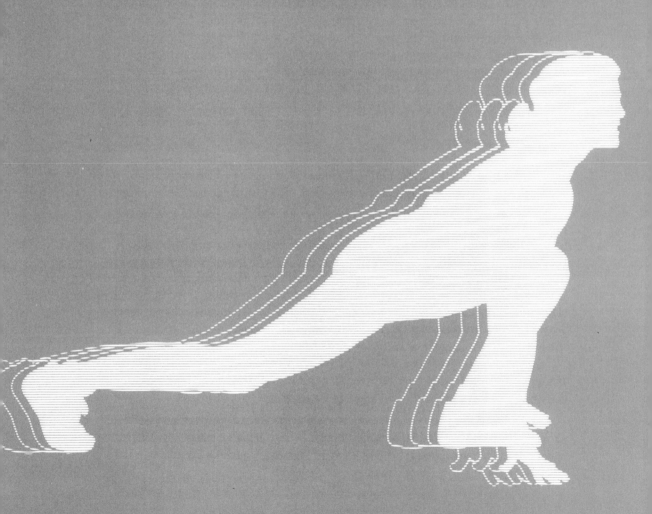

*One day our Cal team* was scheduled to play a match at courts about an hour from the Berkeley campus. One of our players was late and I insisted we wait for him. We all arrived late and harried for the match and had to dispense with our usual pre-match stretching routine. We didn't play well that day. After the match, the players complained, "It was your fault, coach. You didn't get us there in time to stretch."

Stretching has become extremely popular in recent years. More and more active people have discovered its benefits. It increases range of motion, prevents injuries, and develops body awareness. Anywhere you see people working out, training, playing various sports—you'll see them stretching. They know that stretching gets their muscles ready for activity.

## Stretch Gently

The recent popularity of stretching is due in large part to Bob Anderson, who wrote the book *Stretching,* and has travelled the country extensively the past 10 years conducting clinics, lecturing, and demonstrating proper stretching methods. I was one of Bob's first pupils in his International School of Stretching in Denver in 1973. I can remember being so frustrated by not being able to reach the positions Bob was demonstrating. While I was straining, Bob said: "Don't strain, you're not competing." He explained that there was no point in comparing my flexibility with anyone else's. The goal was to stretch *my* muscles gently and gradually improve *my* flexibility. Even though I couldn't get my head on the floor sitting spread-legged, I was getting a lot out of the stretch by working toward that.

Stretching isn't a sport. It's an activity that's necessary for all sports. It's a gradual shifting of gears. In Bob's words, stretching " . . . is a way of signaling your muscles they're about to be used."

Stepping onto the tennis court is a sudden change of pace and scene from sedentary activity. Stretching helps us to bridge that gap, to shift from whatever we've been doing to being ready to play. The 5 to 10 minutes it takes to stretch is time well invested.

# General Stretching Tips

*No pain:* You should never feel any pain when stretching.

*No bouncing:* It can tear muscle fibers.

*Easy does it:* After starting with a slow easy stretch, gradually extend the position further and stretch your muscles more. Go by how it feels. Some days you will stretch farther than others. Listen to your body.

*No comparisons:* You're not competing. Every person's body is different, with different degrees of tightness in various muscles. Stretch your own muscles so you'll be ready to play well and without injury.

*Stretch after playing:* After playing, go through the same stretches to relax tight muscles, improve circulation and wind things down. This will do a great deal to eliminate any soreness the next day.

# Tennis Stretches

On the following two pages are stretches I have worked out over the years, especially designed for tennis players. If you've done any yoga you will notice the similarity of many of these to yoga postures. If you have any particular problem areas not covered by these positions, see *Stretching* (listed in Bibliography, p. 186).

I have my team players start stretching at the top of their bodies and work down. They generally spend at least 10 minutes stretching before practice and matches. These stretches are done before taking the court to warm up. You may want to take longer, or some days you may have time only for an abbreviated version of the routine. But never skip stretching altogether. It's vitally important for your body, as well as your game.

*Stretch for Strength . . . Some physical therapists now believe that stretching not only warms you up for exercise but actually makes the muscles stronger.*

# Tennis Stretches

These are stretches that should be done both before and after playing.

*Before playing*, to:

● Loosen up.

● Give your muscles advance warning they're about to be used.

● Avoid injuries.

*After playing*, to:

● Relax.

● Take out any kinks you get while playing.

● Minimize the soreness that often follows a hard workout.

Stretch in each position until you feel a *slight* muscle tension. Hold this position for 10 to 20 seconds, then stretch slightly farther for another 10 to 20 seconds. With all these exercises that show stretching either the right or left side (or arm or leg), stretch the opposite side as well.

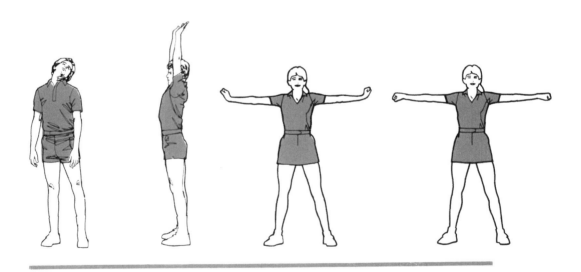

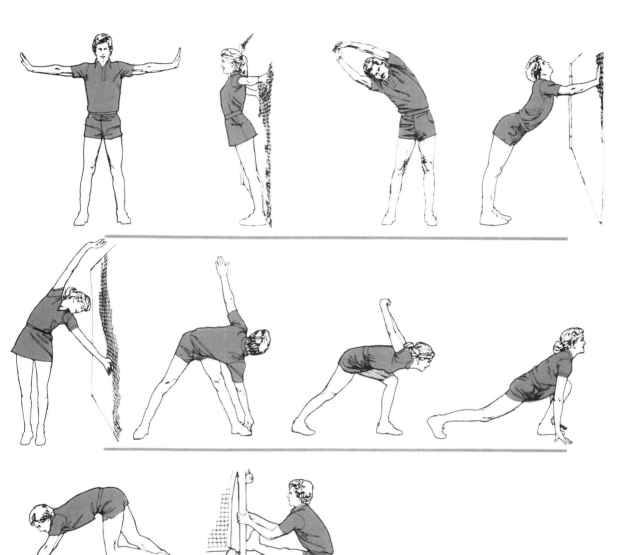

## Remember:

- No pain.
- No bouncing.
- Take it easy.
- Breathe slowly and deeply. □

**Dynamic Scything** . . . *The concept of using your whole body in physical activities isn't limited to tennis. I had explained the concept of using your whole body in tennis to a friend of mine who is an avid gardener. He later told me that when he was scything some grass that spring, he thought of what I said and started using his hips, bending at the knees, winding up and unwinding—rather than just using his arms as he swung the scythe. "It was a much smoother action and I didn't get tired as soon." He was transferring some of the strain to his legs, hips and shoulders and involving his whole body in the scything action.*

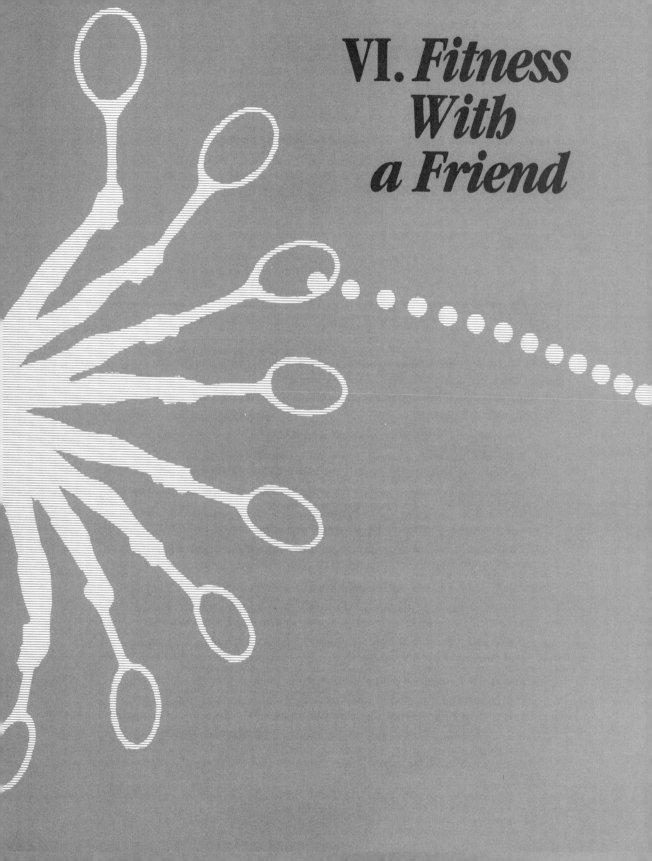

# VI. *Fitness With a Friend*

*It's much more fun* to work out with a partner. Regardless of your level of play, a workout partner can help you improve and be a stimulus to greater activity. There are no secret formulas—you need only the desire to help and a willingness to share the effort of hard work. And if you have found a partner who is willing to drill and practice with you, you have also found a true friend.

## You Don't Have to Be of Equal Skill

Skill is much less important than willingness to help. You can get an excellent workout with someone of less—or more—skill. If you're playing with someone who can't return your shots well enough to give you a good workout, here are some ideas:

● *Alternate workouts:* Your partner stands at the net with a basket of balls and hits you the shot you want to work on. This is a real sacrifice because the person at the net will be getting no exercise. He or she will give you a workout for 10 minutes and then you'll switch.

● *Pick a spot for every ball:* Your practice partner is at the net and you're rallying. You hit your partner one low forehand volley, then a high backhand, then a low backhand. You concentrate on hitting to a specific spot, not just somewhere over the net.

● *Pick your partner's better side:* I was in the backcourt working out with a fairly good player recently. My partner's backhand was his best shot, so in order to work on my own shots, I hit every ball to his backhand. He didn't miss, which was fine with me, since I wanted that ball to come back every time.

● *Put more demands on your shot* (rather than hitting it just anywhere on the court): Hit some cross-court forehands; make your goals very specific and be demanding. Hit the ball deeper than you normally would, or close to the sideline. Stay down on the ball longer and vary your spin.

## *Goals in Practice Matches*

I tell our Cal players they can play practice matches to win as quickly as possible, or just to enjoy being outdoors and improving their suntans; but to work on fitness and becoming better all-around players, they should have goals with each and every shot.

On *groundstrokes* they can have one of these goals each time they hit the ball:

- Staying down with the ball.
- Moving into the ball.
- Hitting a "heavy" ball (ball staying on the strings).
- Keeping the ball deep.
- Disguising direction.
- Varying spin.

On *volleys* a goal might be:

- Penetration.
- Movement after a first volley.
- Hitting short angle volleys with the same preparation as deep volleys.

These are their goals for the day, not for 6 to 4 victories. If they have worked hard to correct a weakness or re-fortify a strength, they have "won the day."

# *Drills*

Drills *can* help you become a better player. You can break your game into its various components and work on whatever needs the most attention. A drill allows you to practice a particular shot or tactic—over and over. If your overhead needs improvement, you can hit 50 of them in a ten minute drill where you might not get a chance to hit 50 in three matches. But drills are a means to an end—that end is to improve your skills.

## Requirements of a Drill

Every drill must be realistic. It must mirror a match situation and it must be done with intensity. Billie Jean King says she drills as if Wimbledon were starting tomorrow. (Don't try to drill with 3 balls. It's too frustrating. Get yourself a basket of balls and don't be afraid to miss.)

## Types of Drills

- *Partner or buddy drills:* In these, your partner does something for the benefit of your game—hits you some specific balls: a lob, a short ball or a backhand volley. Hit them anywhere you want—not necessarily to your partner. You then return the favor.

- *Match play drills:* These drills simulate a playing situation: for example, a cross-court rally drill, a serve and volley drill, a short ball and volley drill. They isolate parts of a playing situation and help create winning sequences of shots.

- *"Overload" drills* (see *Supershape*, p. 162): In these drills the pace is faster than in normal play. An example is the volleyball drill of the Japanese Olympic team where the coach stands 5 to 10 feet from his players and smashes balls at them, one after the other—and the players have to dive and recover. Overload drills can be with one partner, as described below, or with two or more partners.

## 3-Speed Drills

You won't want to go full-out every day. Some days you'll be tired and just not feel like pushing it. Other days you'll feel charged and energetic and want to get a hard workout. You can vary the intensity of your drills accordingly: first gear, or taking it easy; second gear, stepping it up; and third gear, or high speed.

## *Three-Speed Cross-Court Drill*

Let's start with one of the most common and popular groundstroke drills. This will be one-on-one where you and your partner simply hit the ball cross-court to each other.

- *First Gear:* Here you stand in the ally and hit cross-court forehands. Take it slow and keep things under control. You won't get much of a workout because you're not moving much, but you can work on your timing, meeting the ball early, and getting it cross-court.

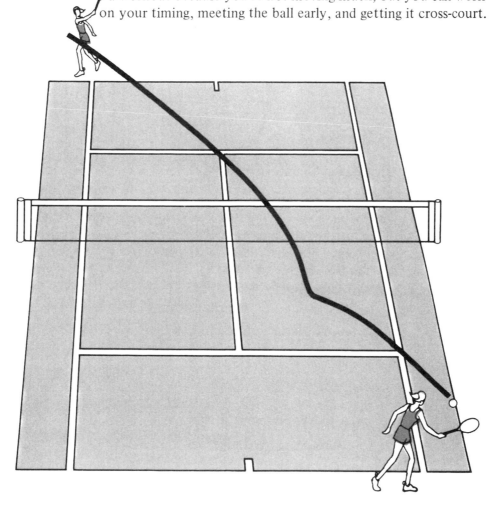

● **Second Gear***:* Put it into second gear and get more of a workout by returning to the middle of the court after hitting each forehand.
Don't just amble back to the middle: Think of springing—exploding—back after hitting the forehand, then exploding back to get the cross-court ball.

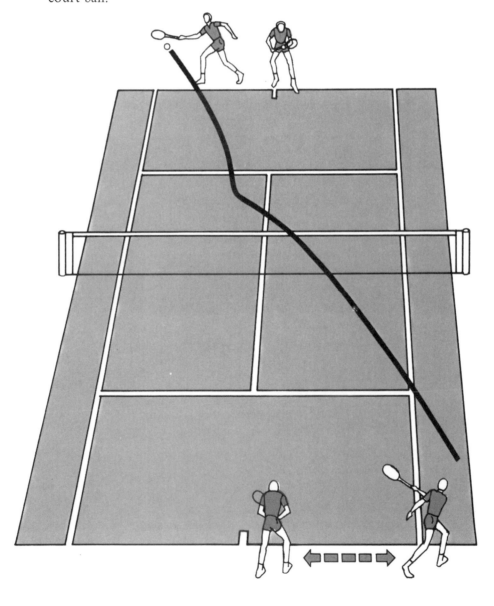

The difference between our fitness drill and the normal cross-court drill is the energy and zest we put into it. Go for a shorter time, but while you are hitting really go after it. Keep in mind that running, reaching, stretching are as much our goals as hitting the ball into the corner.

● *Third Gear:* Let's jazz up the drill even more. Your partner is going to help you with your forehand and later you're going to help her with some aspect of her game that needs special attention. (Both of you can't do this drill at once.) She takes a bucket of 20 to 30 practice balls and hits them to your forehand, from up at the net, from mid-court and the backcourt. She gives you little time to recover. She varies speed, spin and depth.

You hit every ball cross-court and after every hit you return as far to the center of the court as you can, with energy and zest. By the time you've hit 2 to 3 baskets of balls this way, not only will your forehand be better, you'll have had a strenuous workout.

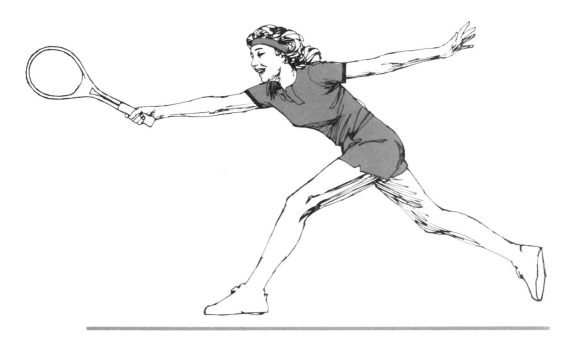

# *Eight Drills*

Our Cal tennis team has about 25 drills. Here are eight of them designed for some of the most common tennis situations and for maximum fitness.

## *Serve & Volley Drill*

*A* serves the ball and comes to the net. *B* lets the ball go by and returns with a ball from the basket. *B* can make it an easy return or rifle it back like Connors. *A* gets the advantage of hitting a tough return since *B* is not actually returning serve.

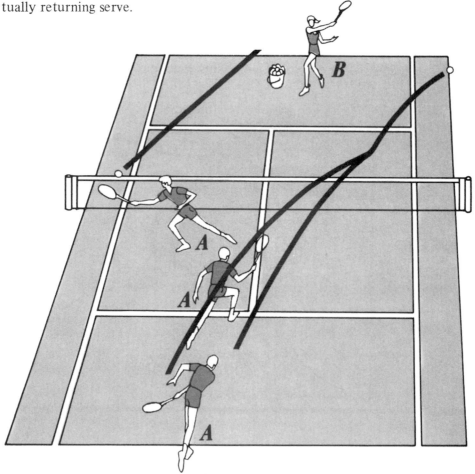

## *Short Ball Drill*

*A* is on the baseline. *B* is on the other side of the net with a basket of balls. *B* hits *A* a variety of short balls. *A* hits them and comes to the net.

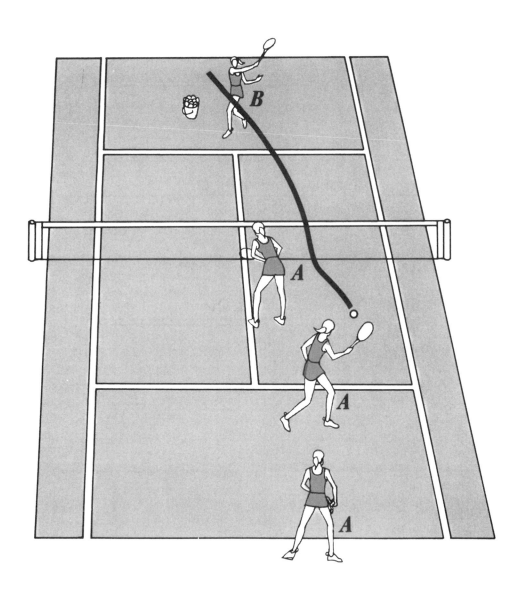

## Australian Little Court Drill

The court is divided right down the middle. Either partner can start the drill by hitting a groundstroke from the baseline and the point is played out using half the court.

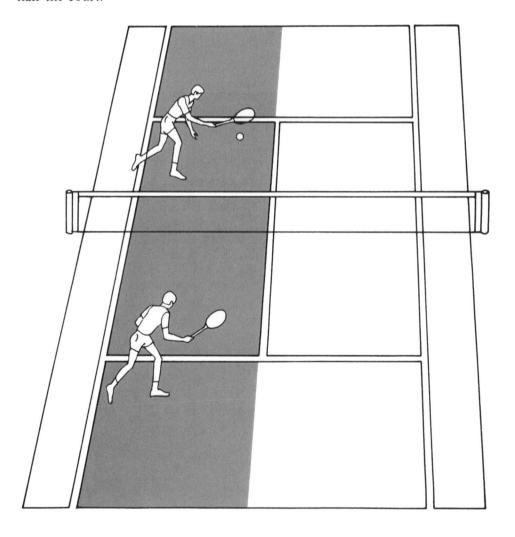

## Short Deep Groundstroke Drill

*A* is on the baseline, *B* is at the net armed with a basket of balls. *B* alternates hitting a short groundstroke, then a deep one to *A*. This gives *A* a strenuous leg workout.

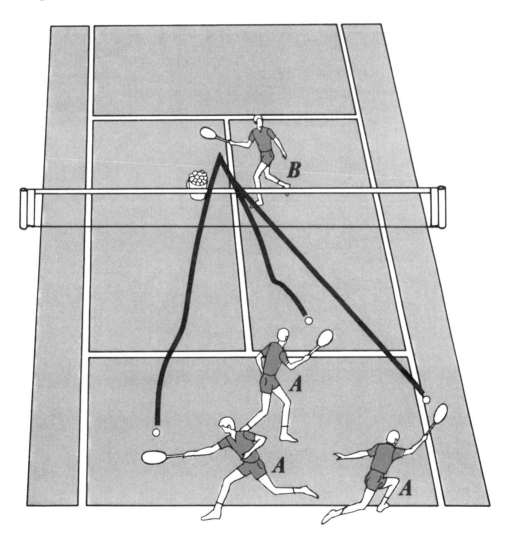

## *No Regard for Your Body Drill*

*A* is either at the baseline or the net. *B* has a basket of balls and hits *A* a continuous stream of balls. *A* has to leap, dive and scramble to get to them.

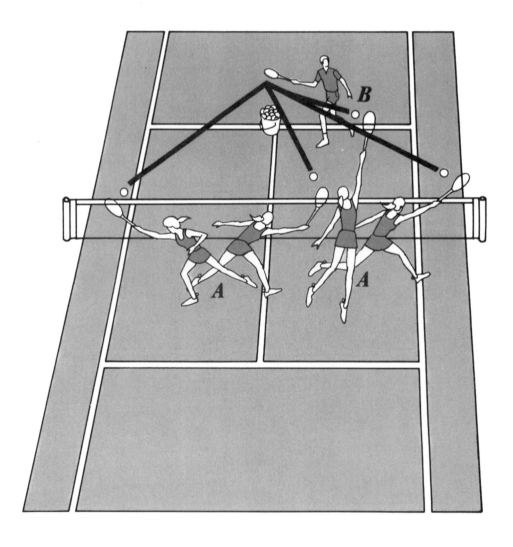

## 25 Balls or Bust Drill

This drill will help you get ready to play a steady baseliner. Both players are in the backcourt. The goal is to hit 25 balls as close to the baseline as you can. Here you try to increase concentration and not get antsy after 5 or 6 balls are hit. If 25 is too hard, start with 5 or 10, etc. . . .

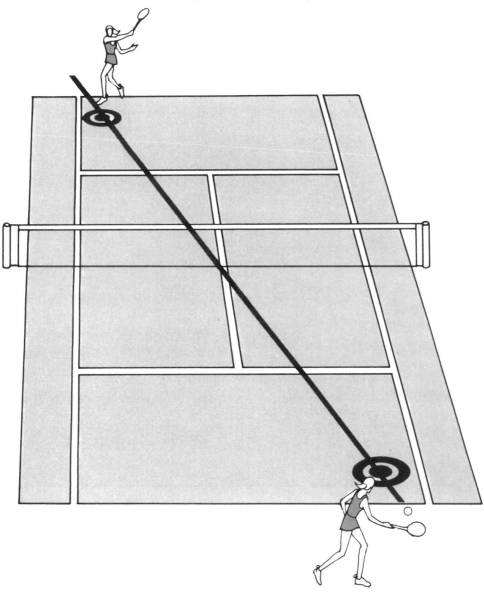

## *Pitching Volley Drill*

You can do this drill anywhere, either on or off the court. *A* has two balls in his hand. From 12 to 15 feet he pitches the balls to *B* underhand. *B* punches the ball with a volley back to *A*. *A* can give *B* a super workout by pitching balls that are barely within his reach. Do this drill to warm up while waiting to get on the court.

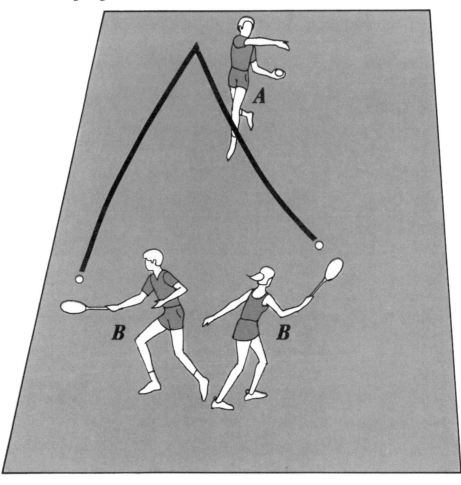

## Hi-Low Volley Dig Drill

Here *A* is at the net. *B* has a basket of balls. She hits one low backhand volley to *A*, then a high forehand volley, then a low forehand volley, followed by a high backhand volley. Five minutes of this is a great stretching and leg workout for *A*.

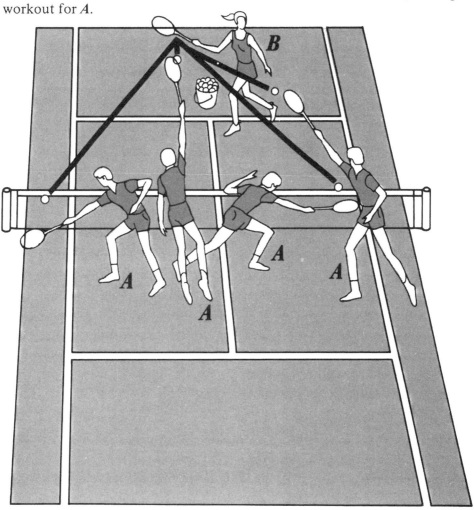

## Beware of Over-Drilling

Drills may mesmerize you into thinking you're doing something extremely well when you're not. In a match you will have to react to a variety of shots and situations, whereas a drill is single-focus. You can get tunnel vision and lose your imagination and spontaneity by drilling too much. Remember, you're not trying to become the world's best driller.□

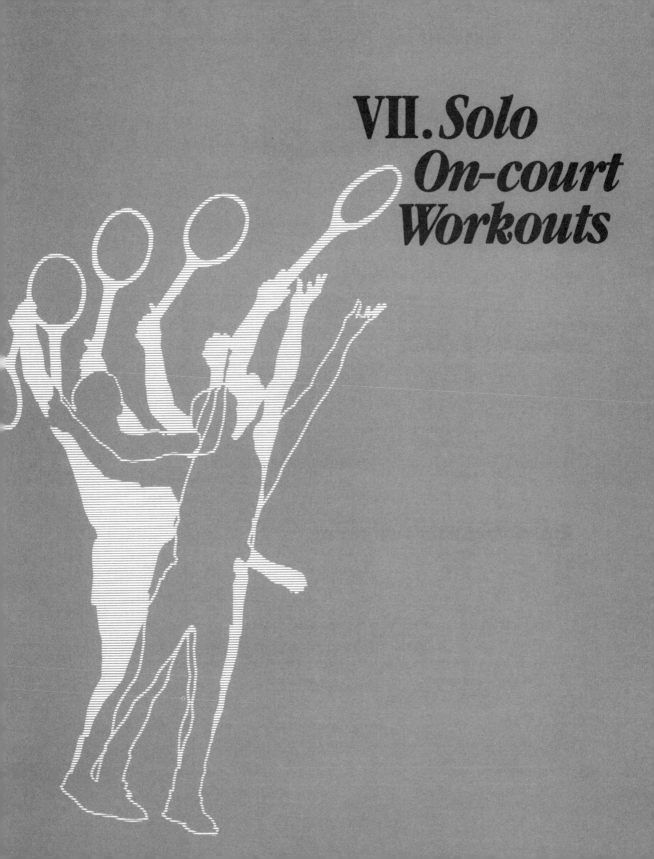

# VII. *Solo On-court Workouts*

- *You suddenly find* you have a spare hour or so to play and there isn't time to find a partner,

- you're stuck on a business trip—you've brought your racket but you can't find anyone to play with, or

- your partner has flaked out on you and you still want to hit some balls.

Where do you go and what do you do?

## Practice Your Shots

Solo workouts don't have to be restricted to the times you can't find a partner. Sometimes a player—even a great player—will want to hit some shots alone. In the 1930's, René LaCoste, the famous French player, came to the U.S. to play an important match with Bill Tilden at Forest Hills. He took a bucket of balls and spent hours dropping the ball and lobbing it to the other baseline. LaCoste won—and partly because he lobbed so well.

## Experiment With Your Serve

If you go on a trip, take along your racket and some balls—even if you don't know any tennis players at your destination. Find a court, do some stretches, warm up, and practice your serve on an empty court. Try some experiments:

- Put more spin on your serve and see how it feels.

- Stand two yards behind the baseline and serve a dozen balls. Then move in and feel how much stronger your serve is when you return to the baseline.

- Serve and sprint to the net.

And usually when you're doing something like this, you'll find that, like magic, someone will materialize and want to start hitting the ball with you.

# *Off the Wall*

When I was about 14, growing up in Cheyenne, Wyoming, I wanted to hit some balls before school every morning. I couldn't get anyone to play with me at that hour and there were no backboards in town, but there *was* a big office building two blocks from our house, next to a parking lot. I would go down at 5:30 in the morning and hit the ball for two hours before school. The janitor ran me off lots of times and finally called my father to complain. But Dad was on my side and convinced the janitor that I really wasn't hurting the granite wall. After that I would play all kinds of imaginary games against the wall. In fact, I won several important Davis Cup matches and national championships in the grey light of dawn in Cheyenne.

Regardless of your skill, the backboard can be a good friend. It will always be there and it will never miss. But just hitting against a backboard can be unproductive and boring, even for the most avid player. Here's how to spice up your backboard practice:

- Draw a line on the backboard with chalk at net level and practice hitting over the net.

- Draw some "x" marks and boxes and see how many times you can hit them.

- If you can control the ball well enough, engage in an imaginary cross-court rally. Hit the ball so the rebound off the wall is a backhand; then hit the backhand so the rebound is a forehand. You can work yourself into a frazzle.

- Serve against the wall, hit overheads against it. . . use your imagination.

*Use Calories Throughout Your Entire Swing . . . Often, all you're concerned with is the final score. If you lose, you feel the match has been a loss. The Aerobic Method emphasizes that if you have run, jumped, stretched and had a good workout, you have accomplished many of your goals. You're going to put out effort; you're not looking for the easy way. The process, the means are important, not just the final score.*

## *Portable Backboard*

Years ago a friend invited me to his tennis club where he had built an ingenious contraption: He had found the plans for a movable backboard in an old tennis book and had built one. A 30 minute workout on a movable backboard is worth an hour and a half with a ball machine, and compared to a ball machine, the portable backboard is cheap, doesn't need electricity or mechanical attention, and doesn't wear out. Unlike a stationary back-·board, it tilts and can give you a much more realistic workout. By adjusting the angle you can simulate any shot. By angling it slightly forward, you can make the ball come to your feet. By slanting it backward, the ball will have lift and you can practice your overhead. This somewhat silent practice partner can do just about everything except bring the balls. □

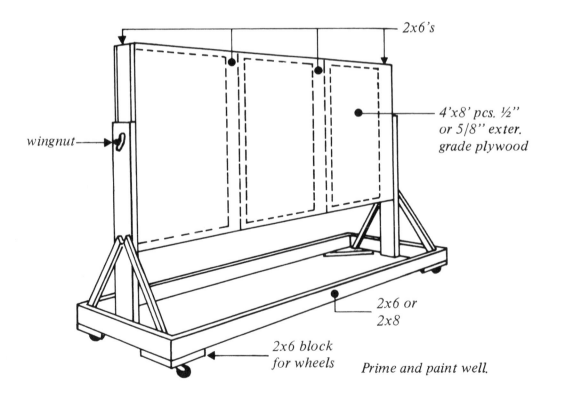

2x6's

4'x8' pcs. ½" or 5/8" exter. grade plywood

wingnut

2x6 or 2x8

2x6 block for wheels

*Prime and paint well.*

# VIII. Off-court Workouts

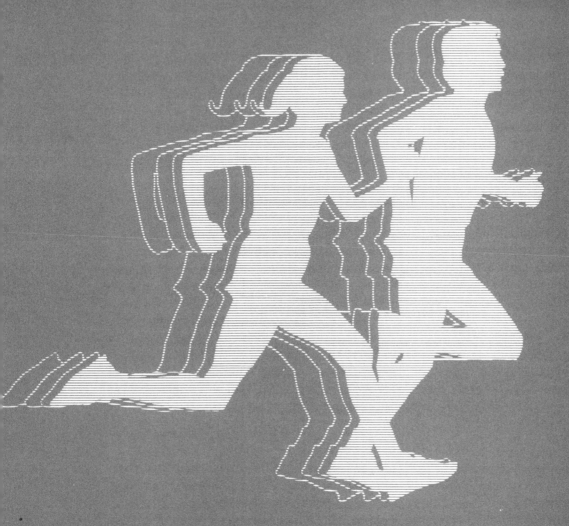

- **Cross-Training**
- **Running**
- **Aerobic Running**
- **Using the Mirror**
- **Aerobic Dancing**
- **Lunch Hour Fitness**

# Cross-Training

**You won't want to play** tennis every day. Moreover, it wouldn't be good for you to play just tennis to the exclusion of other sports and activities. Concentrating on just one sport can lead to muscular imbalance (plus a warped mind). You tend to work on the same muscle groups over and over to the exclusion of others. Bicyclists tend to have huge quadriceps, tennis players over-developed hitting arms, distance runners strong hamstrings and calf-muscles. This kind of specific overdevelopment often leads to muscle damage and poor alignment.

In recent years, trainers and some coaches have begun to emphasize the value of *cross-training,* or engaging in a number of sports to become a better balanced athlete. Combining other sports with your tennis playing will give you a greater overall muscular balance, help prevent injuries and make you a better tennis player. The change of pace will also be refreshing and stimulating. Running, swimming, bicycling, aerobic dancing and cross-country skiing are all excellent aerobic conditioners.

Obviously, Alberto Salazar, the 1982 winner of the Boston Marathon, is in super shape. But in order to run faster, he recently added bicycling and swimming to his training regimen. In the following pages, we'll discuss some basic off-court workouts that will compliment your tennis workouts. Then in the chapter *Supershape,* p. 162, we'll cover more advanced and strenuous workouts like those our Cal team players use.

**Burn It Up** . . . *Your goal is not to conserve energy so you can play all day long, but to **use** energy and get a workout during that limited time you have on the court.*

# *Running*

Running can play a big role in an *Aerobic Tennis* program. You don't need a court, a partner, or any equipment other than good shoes. You can run when you're travelling and at practically any time of the day. Running, the most popular form of aerobic exercise, is one of the best ways to improve your endurance, your strength and your heart and lung capacity. Why don't all tennis players run? For two reasons. There's danger of injury. You're already pounding on a hard court; then to jog on a hard surface may be asking too much of your knees, ankles and feet. And secondly, many players simply find running boring. They think of it as a mere exercise, as a chore.

The danger of injury can be minimized by properly stretching before and after your run, by warming up, by not overdoing it, by wearing the right shoes and by running on soft surfaces whenever possible. And the monotony of running can be relieved by putting some tennis (or spice) into your running. We want to simulate tennis moves and the fatigue you would feel in a match. At the same time we want to add some variety and have some fun.

## *Hop and Jump*

Leg strength is a necessary part of good tennis. The stronger your legs, the more balls you'll get to. Slow down while running to hop forward on one leg 10 times, then on the other. You'll be amazed at the demands on your strength and balance. (Start with 3 or 4 times; work up to 10 or more.) Then try it sideways or backwards, suddenly leaping up to put away that imaginary overhead. Of course, you may not want to do this on the main drag; if your neighbors look out the window and see you running along, then jumping in the air, arm extended, they may think you've played one too many sets in the hot sun.

## *Push Off*

In tennis you don't just run straight ahead; you make a lot of lateral moves. Try pushing off from side to side while you're running. This works well on a sidewalk or a wide path; instead of running down the middle, push and lunge from one side to another—like the movements you make when coming to the net and reaching for a wide volley.

## *Run Sideways and Backwards*

You'll have to run sideways along the baseline. You have to stay low, keep your balance and shuffle your feet quickly. Try some of these movements while running. In the same point, you may have to run backwards and leap for an overhead. At the risk of onlookers thinking you're a bubble off-center, put 10 of these backward sprints into your running routine.

## *Bend for Low Volleys*

When you see a wide spot in the path ahead, come to a stop, knees bent like a shortstop's ready position. Imagine a ball to your right or left and leap to cut off the shot.

# *Aerobic Running*

The word *aerobic* is by now familiar to everyone concerned with fitness. It means, literally, "with oxygen." In practice, it refers to a variety of exercises—running foremost—that stimulate heart and lung activity long enough to improve cardio-vascular fitness and thereby affect changes in the body.

Dr. Kenneth Cooper's best-selling book *Aerobics,* written in 1968, lays out a program of vigorous exercises for 12 to 20 minutes a day during which you sustain a heart rate geared to your age and physical condition. To use this system you must learn how to measure your heart rate.

## Heart Rate at Rest

This is one good indicator of your general fitness. Locate your pulse like this:

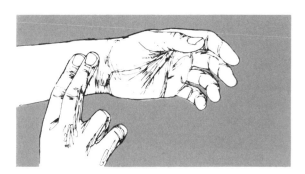

Once you have a steady beat, time the beats for ten seconds with a second hand. Multiply this by six and you have your heart rate at rest. Or measure for 15 seconds and multiply by four.

Once you begin exercising, the heart increases its rate of beating to supply oxygen to the muscles. The more intensively you work out, the harder your heart works and the faster it beats.

**Look For Defeats**... *Look for players who can beat you. This is the way to improve.*

### *Heart Rate While Running*

In strenuous exercise you should have a "target zone" where you exert your-self enough so your heart beats at 70% to 85% of its maximum attainable rate for 12 to 20 minutes, 3 to 4 times a week. A rule of thumb is to sub-tract your age from the figure 220 to get your maximum heart rate. Then take 70% to 85% of that as your target zone. Check your pulse as you run. If you are just starting, stay at the low (70%) end of the zone and gradually increase to the 85% range. You may also want to monitor your pulse while playing tennis to make sure you are running hard enough and using your body to the maximum. After you've practiced this often enough, you'll get to know by just how hard you're breathing when you're in the target zone, and you won't have to keep checking your watch and counting.

*Note: Anyone with high blood pressure, or who is overweight, or has had a heart problem or a family history of heart disease, should consult a doctor before taking part in strenuous aerobic exercise.*

## *Using the Mirror*

Movie and video technology have been a boon to modern sports. Every college football team videotapes their weekly scrimmages and analyzes them the next day. Coaches have found that athletes learn much quicker by seeing themselves in action than by having someone tell them about their perform-ance. Seeing is believing.

I remember vividly one of my first tennis lessons. The pro was trying to show me how to get my racket down below the ball. I couldn't understand this because my racket was below the ball, or so I thought. During a back-swing he shouted, "Stop!" He ran across the court, grabbed my arm and told me to look back and see where the racket was. I was shocked; it was at shoulder level.

Many of us have misconceptions about our racket and body position. If you could see yourself, you'd surely be surprised by some of the things you're doing. If you have access to videotape or home movies, by all means use them. But if you don't, try using a mirror. The mirror can dispel many illusions; you may think you're bending your knees and the mirror may show only a slight flex. Or you may think your wrist is laid back when it's straight as a board.

A pupil will say to me: "That doesn't feel comfortable." But if he can see in a mirror how mechanically unsound that "comfortable" feeling is, he'll be on his way to changing that stroke.

## *Where the Mirror Can Help*

- Position of racket face in backswing.

- Position of racket face at time of hit.

- Position of body at various stages of stroke.

- Overall body balance during preparation and follow-through.

- How to get more bend, reach and stretch.

## *Playing by the Book*

When I was 12, I started playing tennis, thanks to our junior high school P.E. teacher, but often there wasn't anyone to play with. Pretty soon I got a book on tennis and I'd lay it open on the table at home and watch myself in the mirror while I practiced. I'd get so involved in watching my strokes that I wouldn't see the pages of the book flip up. Whack! Off would fly a page as I cracked back that imaginary groundstroke.

# Aerobic Dancing

*"Reach, 2,3,4,5,6,7,8*
*Stretch, 2,3,4,5,6,7,8*
*Push, 2,3,4,5,6,7,8*
Work that body. . .
Every mornin' when we wake
to make up for that piece of cake
we ate last night, we do what's right, all right.
Throw our arms up in the air,
one foot here and one foot there. . ."

*Work That Body* - Paul Jabara/Diana Ross/Ray Chew*

Aerobic Dancing, Dancercise, a Jane Fonda Workout . . . whatever it's called, this exciting fusion of hard calisthenics with good-time music has hundreds of thousands of devotees across the nation reaching, stretching, pushing and jumping to the beat. It has opened up the world of fitness for many thousands who might otherwise never have embarked on an exercise program.

When I was in high school, I always enjoyed P.E. but detested the calisthenics—they were so boring. Much of the activity in aerobic dancing consists of these same or similar exercises but—set to music. What a difference! The music provides the rhythm and an enjoyment of movement that stimulates you to push a little harder and work a little longer.

Our Cal team attends an aerobic dance class several nights a week. After each session the players feel exuberant and energized, rather than fatigued. One of our players, Randy Nixon, worked very hard at aerobic dance. His agility, speed and endurance all improved tremendously during the season and he became our number one player and an All-American. At least part of this came from the way he worked out at aerobic dancing.

* (c) Songs of Manhattan Island Music Co./Rossville Music/Ray-Han Music.

There are many exciting moves in tennis that can be incorporated into a dancersize program. The split steps, the lunges, the leaps, the leg shuffle, etc. are all very similar to tennis movements.

Aerobic dancing has other advantages. Classes often are held at night, so you can get exercise even after you leave your job. All you have to do is show up for the class and you're guaranteed a stimulating workout. The music, the people, and the teacher insure that you'll stretch and work your muscles and get your heart beating strongly. And when you're in good shape you'll want to play more tennis. You won't tire as easily and you'll play a more active game.

Now try taking some of that rhythm and energy onto the court with you. On court the tune is, "I want to move—I want to bend—I want to hit the ball—I want to get some exercise."

# *Lunch Hour Fitness*

If there's a gym nearby, or courts, or a place to run, you can practice any of the techniques we discussed on your lunch hour. Or just take a long brisk walk, breathing deeply; this will do a lot more for you than just sitting and eating. Stop to stretch a little at each corner. Try walking up stairs some times instead of taking the elevator. . . take your pulse and see how much aerobic exercise you can get inside that office building. Use your imagination and think of ways to move and be active during your lunch break. □

***Losing Isn't Everything*** . . . *Years ago, I was watching a friend playing a match. I'd never seen him play before and I noticed that after each point he won, he'd mumble "23 . . . 22 . . . 21 . . . ." I was bewildered and asked another friend what was going on. It turned out that Jack was counting how many more points he needed to win the set. What agony!*

*Certainly we all enjoy winning, but what you're going to get out of this game is the carry-over of fitness and fun. These things will be available to you throughout your entire tennis career—for the rest of your life.*

*Everyone loses sometimes. I've certainly lost. My best loss was to Arthur Ashe in 1963, when he wiped me out in the finals of a Detroit tournament, 6-3, 6-2. It was painful that day, yet as I look back now, this loss is still a highlight of my tournament-playing years.*

# IX. *Supershape*

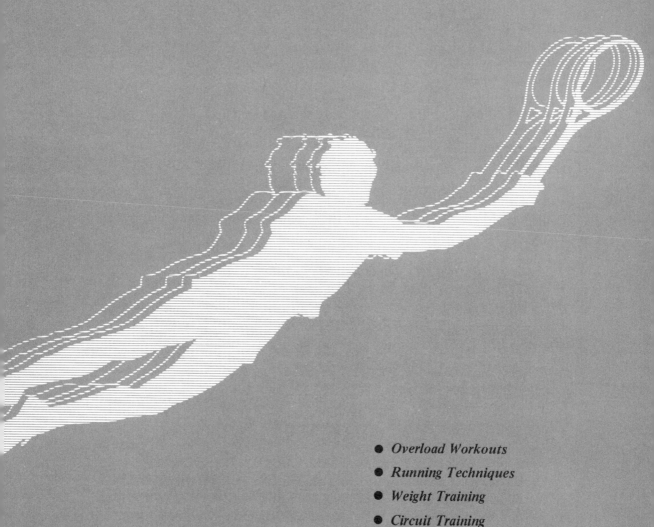

- *Overload Workouts*
- *Running Techniques*
- *Weight Training*
- *Circuit Training*
- *"Go for the Burn"*
- *Triathlons*
- *Take a Break*

*Not too many years ago,* the marathon was thought of as a super endurance feat—one that was performed every four years in the Olympics by extraordinary athletes. Now—in 1983—over 300 marathons will take place across America. Over 16,000 runners started in the New York City marathon in October, 1982. (13,746 finished.) *Supershape* is no longer the province of a few select athletes; people everywhere are uncovering and developing latent athletic ability.

As you play *Aerobic Tennis* you'll find yourself getting in better and better condition. You'll be playing more sets and you'll be taking longer runs. You'll have more endurance, more strength and power. You'll be wanting more exercise and be looking for further challenges. If you're approaching supershape—and you will know—you may want to try out some of the following techniques used by top players in their training schedules. They'll help you move from the zone of good shape to supershape, and help you down the road to becoming an even better tennis player.

*Even if you are in very good physical condition, work into these routines progressively. Push yourself, but don't rush or strain. If you have any questions about your condition or ability to handle highly strenuous activity, consult your doctor before attempting any of the exercises in this section. Train, don't strain.*

# *Overload Workouts*

Athletes have been using the overload principle to increase strength, endurance, and performance for years. One of the earliest written accounts of the overload principle comes from Homer's *Iliad,* where boxers trained with leaded weights on their hands, and runners ran with weighted shoes. Most modern athletes use these principles. Swimmers tie their legs together to make their arms work more. A runner will practice running faster than his race pace. Football linemen push massive blocking dummies around the field.

Ellsworth Vines, a U.S. Open and Wimbledon Champion in the 1930's, spent one winter working with a net 6 inches higher than normal. It took much more effort for him to get down under the ball and lift it—he was overloading. When he resumed playing with a normal net, it was much easier. It's like a batter swinging two bats, then stepping up to the plate with one. He feels like Hercules. Or a runner training by running up hills. When he runs on flat land, it's a lot easier.

In a normal match you may hit three cross-court forehands, then a short ball, then come to the net. The point then stops while you pick up the ball and rest. In our strenuous overload workouts, there are no rests; everything is in high gear. You may hit 15 to 20 cross-court forehands before hitting a short ball and coming to the net. Your partner will be feeding you a continuous series of balls and you'll be hitting a non-stop stream of shots, with no rest to grumble about misses. These rapid-fire sessions give you the chance to work on your fitness and at the same time improve your stroking ability.

## *Two-on-One*

The most stimulating overload workout is the two-on-one workout popularized by the Australians. Here, two players give one player an intense workout. There are no out balls—every ball is played. 10 minutes of working out like this will do more for your fitness than playing two casual sets.

The varieties of this two-on-one type drill are numerous. Here are a couple:

- Single player at net, two players in backcourt. They pelt her with volleys and lobs, making sure she can reach every ball, but making her dig for each one.

- Switch around: The single player is on the baseline, working hard at keeping his groundstrokes deep to the two players on the baseline. They keep him digging and hustling after each ball. After 5 to 10 minutes, switch—the single player can get a rest as one of the doubles workout partners.

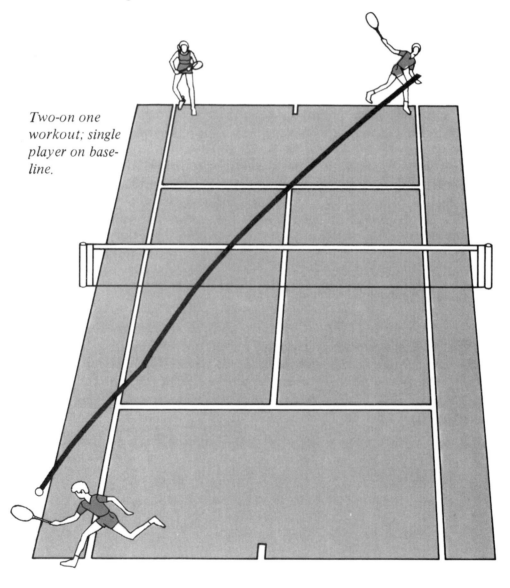

*Two-on one workout; single player on base-line.*

## *Three or More*

You can drill this way when court usage is limited. The objective is to give one or more players a very intensive workout. Some examples:

- Three servers, one returner. Play out each point, then rotate servers.

- One feeder, one backcourt player, two at net. The feeder starts by hitting the ball to one backcourt player. He then tries to pass or lob the two players at the net.

- One feeder in the backcourt, three taking short balls and playing out the point. The feeder hits a short ball to one of the players in the backcourt, who then hits a short ball and comes to the net. The feeder then hits him two volleys and an overhead. Then the back-court players switch.

# *Running Techniques*

## *Time Yourself*

Get a digital wristwatch with a stopwatch. If you run the same route a few times a week, time yourself at key intervals . . . when you reach the park, at the crest of the hill, the house at the corner, etc. Try to improve your times. It will give you some extra incentive when running. And sometimes run *without* the watch, just for the fun and exhilaration of it.

*Use 9/10 of Your Power & Speed . . . A track coach once told his team, "Run this race at 9/10 speed." Then he said, "O.K., now run full out, hard as you can go." He timed them both ways. They ran faster at the 9/10 speed. Why? Because they were more relaxed. Think of this when you're playing.*

## *Runner's Smorgasbord*

Short bursts of speed are needed in a match. After a serve, you'll have to sprint to the net. Or you may be at the net and have to turn and run down a lob. To do this over the length of a long match takes speed, agility and endurance. Intersperse your running with 20 to 30 yard sprints where you pick a tree or telephone pole and sprint for it. When you reach it, don't stop, but slow to medium speed, then to a jog. These three changes of pace are refreshing and add some variety to your running. This is a Swedish runners' training technique called *fartlek*. You push the body hard with untimed efforts over whatever challenges are available: hills, wooden paths, sand at the beach. Then after pushing hard, you take it easy, slowing it down in stages.

## *Enter a Race*

Don't start with a marathon, but try a casual neighborhood 10 kilometer or shorter race. "Social" running can be a lot of fun. You'll discover that you push yourself harder than you thought possible when you're in a race. Don't be reluctant to enter because you're afraid you'll lose. There will be runners of all levels. You don't have to tie yourself in knots over excelling, but it's something to work toward, enjoy while you're doing, and think about afterwards.

# *Weight Training*

So often we think of tennis as purely a game of skill. But it's also a game of strength. In the 1950's, Harry Hopman, the Australian Davis Cup coach, was the first well-known and respected world class coach to use weight training for tennis players. With the help of a heavy weight training program, he helped both Margaret Court and Frank Sedgeman become world class players. In recent years, players of all sports—once they've overcome the myth of becoming muscle-bound—have discovered that weight training can improve not only their strength and endurance, but flexibility as well.

A stronger player is a better player. Chip Hooper was a junior college tennis player in California before he went to the University of Arkansas in 1979. There he became friends with a number of football players and they encouraged him to start a weight training and strength building program. With the help of these training methods, Chip ended up the no. 1 seed in the 1981 NCAA championships and is now among the top 25 players in the world. He attributes much of his success to weight training.

There are two basic types of training: free weights and machines. By free weights we mean barbells and dumbbells. Machines like Nautilus or Universal are substantially different, offer heavy resistance throughout a full range of movement, and can be used very specifically to work out individual muscles.

## Free Weights

Don't start a free weight lifting program without considering what areas of your body need strengthening. Some people will need more upper body strength, others more work in the legs. On the other hand, a player who is already strong may not want the additional bulk that weight training might add.

*Note: A good coach or instructor is important. Technique is critical and you don't want to use too much weight and cause muscle injury. Special care should be given to the back. Never lift free weights without a weight lifting belt—a thick leather strap that supports your back—and a training partner.*

## Advantages of Free Weights

Although weight machines have become very popular, the current trend among strength training coaches is a return to free weights. The overall body strength from gripping, lifting and balancing a free bar gives the athlete greater overall muscular, tendon and ligament strength than do machines. Free weights will do more for your balance and coordination and will help with your concentration and timing, which will be valuable in all sports. Al Vermeil, the innovative strength training coach (formerly with the San Francisco 49'ers), is a firm believer in cross-training with lots of overloading techniques, from using medicine balls, to jumping *off* boxes, to jumping *on* boxes, to lifting weights. He prefers free weights over the machines because of the coordination, strength and balance they require.

## Tips on Lifting

● Combine lifting with playing tennis but, in general, don't take a day off from playing to lift weights. Combine a tennis workout with a weight session. Out Cal players generally lift weights *after* a tennis workout.

● Stretch the muscles used before and after lifting.

● Always warm up carefully before lifting.

● Always finish a complete range of motion when you lift.

● Train, don't strain.

*A Weak Shot to the Right Place* . . . *Bill Tilden, in* **How To Play Better Tennis,** *said that the most beautifully executed shot to the wrong place is not nearly as desirable as a weak shot to the right place.*

# *Some Tennis Weight Training Exercises*

The following exercises are particularly helpful for players who lack upper body strength. Although traditionally a male-oriented activity, weight lifting has recently become popular with women. Women players will find they can control the ball much better after just a few weeks of these exercises. And remember, weight training is a supplement to playing tennis, not a substitute. Be conservative. *Under*-do it at first. Use weights that give you resistance but do not cause strain.

### *Wrist Curls*

*For hands,
wrists, fingers:
Roll your
wrists
up and down.*

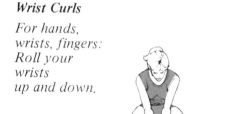

### *Triceps*

*Be sure
to keep
elbows close
to your side
and isolate
tension in
triceps.*

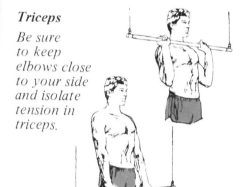

### *Barbell Curl*

*For forearms and biceps:
Lower and raise arms
slowly with complete
extension and stretch.*

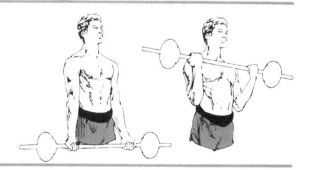

*Note: Wear a belt and have a partner for shoulders, chest and leg exercises.*

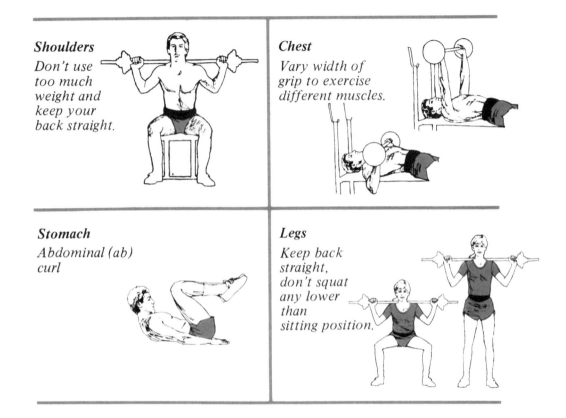

**Shoulders**
Don't use
too much
weight and
keep your
back straight.

**Chest**
Vary width of
grip to exercise
different muscles.

**Stomach**
Abdominal (ab)
curl

**Legs**
Keep back
straight,
don't squat
any lower
than
sitting position.

# Balancing Your Left Arm

Your hitting side is obviously getting much more muscle development. You
can compensate for one-sidedness in a gym. Do exercises where your left
hand (if you're right-handed) has to do its share of work. Use dumbbells and
do arm presses where the left hand has to hold on to the weight by itself.
Always stretch that side well.

## *Weight Machines*

The machines are simple and safe and you can get a good workout. Nautilus machines are particularly good for tennis players because they include stretching and controlled resistance through a full range of motion. You can isolate muscles to be worked on and it's easier to work just your upper body than it is with free weights.

Both Billie Jean King and Arthur Ashe used Nautilus machines in recovering from injuries. They both went through the Nautilus routines, got in some cardio-vascular work to build up their endurance, and went back to play even better tennis.

## *Power Without Weights*

If you look at Herschel Walker, Georgia's great All-American running back, in a swim suit you'd swear he spent three hours a day in a gym, lifting heavy weights and using a Nautilus machine. Yet to everyone's surprise, Herschel does none of this. His workout routine? Pushups, sit-ups (abdominal curls), windsprints and swimming. He's built like Hercules, yet he uses no hardware. So even though weights are now thought of as being synonymous with strength, power and a muscular look, they're not necessary. This is good news for people who don't have easy access to a gym or who don't want to bother with the weight routines. You can build muscle without pumping iron.

# *Circuit Training*

In circuit training you run on a set route. As you run, you stop along the way to perform various exercises, overloading your muscles when you are aerobically stressed. You exercise in the middle of a run while you are breathing hard and your heart is pumping strongly.

Circuit training will increase strength and improve oxygen capacity. The two work together. If you stop to do pushups while your heart is pumping hard, you can't get much oxygen to your arms and chest muscles because it's going to the rest of your body. This makes your muscles tight and you have to work harder to do the pushups. This is a form of overloading and strengthens you much more than pushups done with a normal pulse rate.

Circuit training is a fine conditioner for tennis, since tennis does not entail only a sustained effort like long-distance running, nor is it comprised solely of short bursts of strength. It's a combination of endurance and strength. Imagine a rally in the 5th set where you hit five groundstrokes, a short ball, two volleys, then a tough overhead; this is circuit training on the court. You can approximate these demands on your body while training on a circuit.

## *Par Courses*

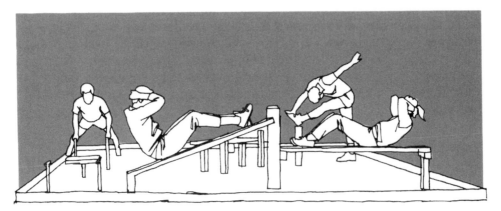

Exercise stations such as these have been set up in various places around the country for circuit training.

# Cal Tennis Circuits

Here is one of the circuits we use in Berkeley. Our players are asked the following questions:

- *Load:* Am I increasing the number of times I do the exercises as my strength increases?

- *Repetitions:* Am I increasing the number of times I do exercises as my fitness increases? (There are limits, of course.)

- *Time:* Am I performing the maximum amount of work in the shortest possible time?

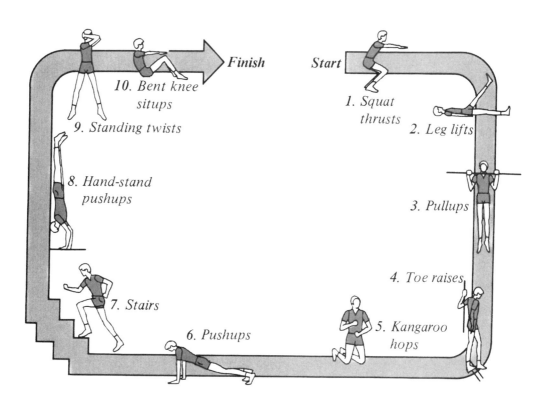

Finish

Start

10. *Bent knee situps*

9. *Standing twists*

8. *Hand-stand pushups*

7. *Stairs*

6. *Pushups*

1. *Squat thrusts*

2. *Leg lifts*

3. *Pullups*

4. *Toe raises*

5. *Kangaroo hops*

## Create Your Own Circuit

If you're not near a specially designed par course, make up your own. Run to the corner and do 20 to 30 pushups, then to the next mailbox and do 30 abdominal curls. Each time around the course try to do a few more push-ups or abdominal curls than the last time. Knee bends, calf raises on the curb, step-ups, toe raises, pushups, ab curls, etc. are easily adaptable to any circuit (see previous page). If you live near a school or playground, there will be many potential exercise stations. Look around, be creative, vary your circuits from day to day and try to have some fun.

## "Go for the Burn"

We talked about the fun and stimulation of aerobic dancing. When you begin aerobic dancing, you have to be careful. The music, companionship and excitement can push you too hard and you can hurt yourself. However, once you've been to enough classes and worked out at other activities enough to get strong, you can "go for the burn," as some of the aerobic teachers say. You push yourself until you feel a burning sensation in the muscles. This means you are exercising that particular muscle extremely vigorously. You can do this in a regular class by just pushing it hard, or you can go to an advanced aerobic class where a 1½ hour session will probably be a tougher workout than anything you could put yourself through. It's important that you learn to distinguish between the burn of overloaded muscles and actual injury. Again, don't strain.

# *Triathlons*

Ten years ago, who would have dreamed there'd be so much interest in running marathons? Now people are looking for further ways to test themselves. Thus the triathlons, which come in various sizes and shapes. Generally they consist of swimming, running and bicycling. The grand-daddy of the triathlons is the *Hawaii Iron Man,* a 2.4 mile swim, a 112 mile bicycle ride, and a 26.2 mile marathon—all done in one day! Obviously, only superbly conditioned athletes are going to try something like that. But now there are more and more scaled-down versions of the *Iron Man* all over the country. For example, Berkeley has a popular triathlon: a 2-K swim in Lake Anza, a 40-K bike ride through the Berkeley hills, and a 10-K run through Tilden Park.

You can make up a triathlon to suit your own training program. A three-sport training session tests and works all the muscles. Running builds up the hamstrings and calf muscles, bicycling works the quadriceps and shin muscles, and swimming works the upper body and most of the major body muscles. You could do a two-mile run, a 500 yard swim (in a pool, a lake, the ocean) and a five-mile bike ride and probably finish it in less than an hour and a half. You'd get a vigorous and balanced workout, enjoy yourself and certainly not be bored.

# *Take a Break*

Finally, don't get so involved with super conditioning you forget to take a day off at least once a week. Once you get in better shape you have to guard against over-training. Spend some time relaxing with friends or family, and do something different. You'll go back to training with rested muscles and with renewed vigor and interest. □

**Look For Challenges** . . . *I once heard Glenn Bassett, coach at UCLA, tell the story of one of his most famous players' disappointment and frustration when his practice opponent missed a shot—the ball didn't come back over the net—and there was no ball to hit. He felt cheated. He had come on the court to play, to hit, to run, to stretch and he couldn't do all this because his opponent missed the ball. How different from the usual frame of mind when playing tennis! We are so often guilty of missing the boat—we generally want our opponent to miss, we want some easy points. When we first started to play, we wanted to be challenged, to work hard and get a good workout. But we soon became so fixated on winning, on technicalities and on image, that we forgot about the real challenges of playing. Try thinking to yourself: "I want that ball to come back . . .," and see what a difference it makes in your practice sessions.*

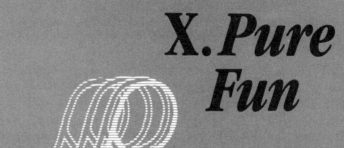

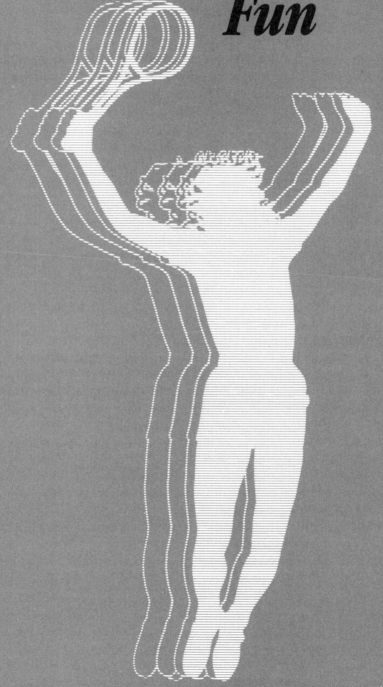

# Exercise, Play and Sport

**Competitiveness, hard work and intensity** are part of any sport. But some days you won't feel like being serious. You'll just want to *play*. You'll want to do something on the court that is spontaneous, relatively unstructured, and where the consequences of failure are not great.

In a recent issue of *The Physician and Sportsmedicine,* Dr. George Sheehan wrote about the difference between exercise, play and sport. *Exercise,* he said, is work. *Play* is pure fun, something we do for the sheer joy of it—no rules, no restrictions. *Sport* is both exercise and play with something at risk—rules.

Sometimes you'll just want to enjoy the sound of the ball hitting the strings. Following are a few games you can play to take a break from intensive workouts, and from the seriousness of matches. They will rekindle your enthusiasm.

## Dinkum

What's amazing about Dinkum is the energy and enthusiasm that go into it. It's played inside the service court and you cannot hit the ball "too hard." Unlike what happens in a match, you *want* your opponent to get to the ball. You play for the sheer pleasure of hitting it. The rules are somewhat hazy, and you can modify them as you please. I can look at you and say, "You hit that ball too hard, that doesn't count. Let's play the point over." And you say, "O.K., fine." It's like playing catch with a child—you throw the ball gently so the child can catch it. In Dinkum you want that ball to come back. You're working on your touch and feel, and having fun. It's like you're teasing each other. You do keep score, but the score is soon forgotten.

Several years ago at the NCAA championships in Athens, Georgia, Elliot Teltscher had been upset in a grueling match in the morning. After the match, he seemed exhausted and discouraged, yet that same afternoon he came out and played Dinkum with a friend—laughing, carrying on and having a great time. I used to think Dinkum was a waste of time, that it would be better to practice your serve. What I didn't understand or appreciate was the enjoyment that players got from it.

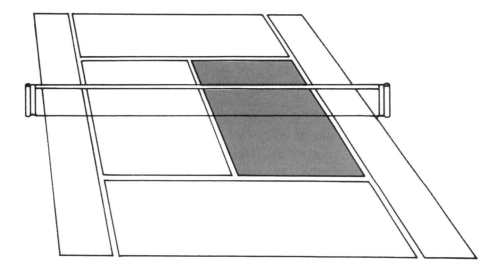

*Boundaries of Dinkum court in color; confining yourself to this zone will develop your touch.*

# 5 O'Clock Ball

At a recent tournament in Los Angeles, our players finished their matches early and, at the suggestion of one player, all met at the deserted courts at 5 o'clock, where they played some of their most enjoyable and best tennis of the year. The matches were very short. You played the best 2 out of 3 games with the winner staying on the court and the loser having to sit it out. The players hated to lose; they would do anything to stay on the court. It was very aggressive tennis, but played in the spirit of pure fun. The first loser had to buy the second loser an Orange Julius, and so on.

# Round the World

This is a similar game, an elimination contest—popular at many tennis camps. You need about 8 or more players. Four line up on opposing sides of the net. The ball is put in play by an underhanded serve and a rally begins. After you hit the ball, you run to the other side of the court, taking your place in line behind the other players. If you miss the ball, you must sit down and a new ball is put into play. When there are only two players left on each side, the rules change: after you hit the ball, you drop your racket, do a 360 degree turn, pick up your racket and hit the next ball. Each time we've had a group play it at a camp, players have had so much fun we've had trouble getting them off the court.

# Rallies

Rallies can be pure fun. There's no score, no one sitting down or left out, and there's no stigma about missing the ball. Rallies are great when you're coming back from an injury or a lay-off. Start out by rallying rather than playing sets. There's no stress and no competitive urge to hit the ball harder. You'll be less likely to strain or pull those unconditioned muscles.

# *Catch-It*

In Athens, Georgia, before the beginning of the NCAA individual men's championships in 1982, I was walking along the backcourts discussing some team business with a sporting goods representative, when University of Michigan coach Brian Eisner stopped us and said, "Come over here, you've got to see this."

His number one player Mike Leach was armed with a racket and was serving against his doubles partner Mark Mees, who had no racket. Mike would serve, Mark would run and catch it, and then try to throw it past Mike to win the point. It was about 100 degrees and the boys were both dripping wet, but the element of pure fun kept them going—they were laughing and joking and carrying on. This interlude of relaxation from the rigors of practice must have helped, for later that week Mike went on to win the NCAA men's singles championship.

# *The Real Fun of Tennis*

All of us who play tennis know how our lives have been enriched by the friends we've made on the court. And when we play tennis with someone we already know, the comraderie of competing and cooperating adds zest and meaning to our friendship.

While we frequently run into characters like Your Friendly Court Hog, Your Opponent the Umpire, or Your Partner the Court General, we also see the best of people on the court. They don't shout or throw temper tantrums, but they're not afraid to show their enthusiasm for the game and their respect for their opponents either. There are no grand gestures, no great emotional demonstrations, and if you tried to describe these qualities after the match, you might have trouble finding the right words. A smile, a friendly gesture, an acknowledgement of a good shot, 100% effort when all is going awry—there is something that sets these players apart.

Richard Evans described what I'm talking about in an excellent article in *World Tennis* in December 1976. Australia and Italy were locked in an inter-zone Davis Cup battle in 1972, with the winner to play Chile for the Davis Cup. Adriano Panatta and John Newcombe were in the middle of the deciding singles match when the ever fiercely partisan Italian crowd started behaving as never before:

> *"Four days this battle had raged with neither team able to establish a commanding lead, but at last, in this fifth and deciding rubber, Italy seemed on the brink of the final breakthrough. It was in the fourth set and Panatta had a break and then his opponent double-faulted, and two points later double-faulted again. Crowds in Rome have been known to clap and cheer an opponent's double-faults. But now something odd happened, something stranger than all the unlikely happenings that had gone before. The crowd started chanting, "New-combe, New-combe." They didn't want him to win, of course, but they were prepared to risk lifting him—as they know a crowd could lift a player—out of his trough of depression, because they liked him and respected him and didn't want to see a great champion humiliated.*
>
> *It had been obvious right from the start that there was this* simpatico *between Newcombe and the Roman crowd. Unlike so many foreign players, Newcombe had never made the mistake of getting uptight about their antics and their fierce favoritism. Instead of scowling at them like an enemy, he had laughed and joked with them and pulled faces and now they were telling him how much they appreciated it. When it was all over, when even the crowd's brief accolade had failed to revive John Newcombe, and Italy won this enthralling inter-zone final by three rubbers to two, we had to pull the kids and even some adults out of the mini-bus one by one as they grabbled for Newcombe's autograph. Not many defeated warriors have been treated so well in Rome."*

Perhaps you'll never have a huge crowd express such appreciation for you exhibiting *that little something extra,* but if one opponent, one spectator, one coach feels it—that will be enough. □

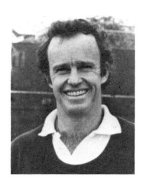

# *About*
# *The Author*

*Bill Wright* grew up in Cheyenne, Wyoming, and started to play tennis when he was 12, and he's been hooked ever since. Between tournaments and coaching, he attended Southern Methodist University in Dallas. While getting his law degree at Denver, he coached there and at Colorado State University. In 1960 he was the Southwest Conference Doubles Champion and Inter-mountain Doubles Champion. In 1963 he was ranked no. 44 in the United States in men's singles. In 1964 he was the coach and captain of the U.S. Junior Davis Cup Team.

Bill practiced law for five years in Los Angeles before returning to tennis full-time as coach at the University of Illinois and director of tennis during the summers at Vail, Colorado.

In 1974 he was ranked no. 7 in the U.S. in the 35-and-older category. That same year he began coaching the men's team at the University of California at Berkeley and for six years his team was in the quarterfinals or higher in the NCAA team championships. He became the vice president of the Intercollegiate Tennis Association in 1976.

In 1978 the NCAA coaches picked him as Coach of the Year. In 1980 the Cal Bears won the national indoor team championships and were runners-up to Stanford in the NCAA championships. In 1982 Bill was named Coach of the Year in the Pac-10 Conference. His coaching at Cal has produced seven all-Americans, all of whom have since turned professional.

From 1987 to 2006, he was men's tennis head coach at the University of Arizona. He was named Region Eight Coach of the Year in 2003 and in 2005. In 2006, he was elected into the Intercollegiate Coach's Hall of Fame, as well as the Colorado Tennis Hall of Fame. During his 27 years as a coach, he accumulated a 373–319 career record.

He and his wife, Bitsy, currently live in Tucson, Arizona.

# *Bibliography*

*Here are brief reviews of eight outstanding tennis books and five books on other aspects of fitness. Almost every book on tennis currently in print is available by mail from the United States Tennis Association, 51 East 42nd Street, New York, N.Y. 10017. They'll send you their list of publications upon request.*

### The Aerobics Program For Total Well Being

By Dr. Kenneth Cooper. M. Evans and Co., Inc., New York, N.Y. 1982.

Cooper brought the word "aerobics" into common usage with his book *Aerobics* in 1968. He followed that with three more aerobics books and now puts together his most recent discoveries and conclusions, some of which may surprise his readers:

1. If you're running more than 3 miles, 5 times a week, you're running for something other than fitness . . . .

2. It's not the total amount of cholesterol in your body that is the health hazard, but rather the lack of a proper balance between two different types of cholesterol . . . .

3. Do your aerobic exercise at the end of the day, just before the evening meal . . . .

4. To *lose* weight, consume your calories by the "25-50-25" rule: 25% at breakfast, 50% at lunch, 25% at dinner. To *maintain* weight, go to 25-30-45.

   Some stimulating conclusions and well worked-out fitness programs from someone who's been involved with aerobics and fitness for some 25 years.

### Arthur Ashe's Tennic Clinic

By Arthur Ashe. Illustrations by Jim McQueen. Tennis Magazine/Simon and Schuster, New York, N.Y. 1981.

In this book you can attend a tennis clinic with Arthur Ashe, the head pro, and have some of the world's best players drop in to show you some of their shots. To simulate a clinic, most of Ashe's tips and advice are presented in illustrations, not words. The exciting color drawings, great diagrams and concise tips make this a real plus for every player. Arthur's strategy and conditioning chapters are good, but his instructions on serve and volley, like his game, are world class. This book, more than any other, shows the great physical demands of tennis. When you see the drawings of the great players hitting the ball, you can almost hear the energy and effort they are putting into each shot.

### How To Play Better Tennis: A Complete Guide to Tactics and Technique
By Bill Tilden, Cornerstone Library, New York, N.Y. 1950.

When one of the greatest tennis players of all time confesses that he was often so discouraged in playing that he had recurring dreams of burning his rackets, you know you are getting a candid view of tennis and how he thinks it should be played. This tennis classic was written over 30 years ago, yet is as useful today as it was in the '50's. It covers hitting the ball, strategy and tactics—clearly and understandably. Throughout the book you sense Tilden's love of tennis and commitment to the game. He urges you not to be impatient, that it takes time to become a good player, but that the time and effort are well worth it. It's a simple book and doesn't overwhelm you with technicalities.

### Improving Your Running
By Bill Squires with Raymond Krise. Stephen Greene Press, Brattleboro, VT. 1982.

This book is probably the next-best thing you could have to a running coach. Bill Squires was a three-time All American runner at Notre Dame and coached Bill Rodgers, Lorraine Moller and Alberto Salazar. There are training programs for "fun runs," 10-K races, 10 mile races and marathons. There are chapters on racing strategy, common injuries, nutrition for the runner, and maintaining your strength.

A few tips:

1. Fluids: The best drink is water.

2. Sleep before a race: Get a good night's sleep two nights before the race. Then you'll be rested enough even if nerves keep you awake the night before.

3. Marathon: Take your last hard workout 12 days before the race. Eat enough to just stay alive until 1½ days before the race. Then load up on the right kind of food. Your last pre-race meal is 16 hours before race time.

4. Runners high: Medical studies have shown that after 25 minutes or so of aerobic exercise, the runner's brain "opens up," inspired by the extra oxygen.

### The Inner Game of Tennis
By W. Timothy Gallwey, Random House, New York, N.Y. 1974.

I remember vividly the impact of Gallwey's book. Players started coming to Vail and began their tennis sessions saying to themselves, "Bounce . . . hit; bounce . . . hit . . . ." They were obviously trying to forget some complicated instructions they'd had and " . . . just let it happen." It certainly made me think about my own teaching methods and whether I was making things too technical and complicated for my players. Gallwey had great faith that once we " . . . let it flow," the ability to hit the ball would be there. If you just could turn off your analytical mind and get over to the right side of your brain, he felt your body and instincts would know what to do. The book is so well written it's hard to put down. There are interesting experiences and observations from Gallwey's teaching years on almost every page. It's easy to see why this book became a best seller and continues to sell today, ten years after it was published.

### Bill Pearl's Keys to the Inner Universe
Bill Pearl Physical Fitness Architects, Pasadena, Calif. 1980.

Bill Pearl, one of the world's top body builders, takes you through every possible weight lifting exercise in this giant compendium. There are exercises for practically every muscle in the body, along with drawings of the different positions. The book covers weight machines—Nautilus and Universal—along with free weights, and goes further than any other book in explaining the science of body building.

### Pancho Segura's Championship Strategy: How To Play Winning Tennis
By Pancho Segura with Gladys Heldman. McGraw Hill Book Co., New York, N.Y. 1976.

Here you can share some strategy sessions with one of tennis' leading gurus. Pancho was such a great player because of his incredible will to win and his analysis of opponents. The book is filled with anecdotes and stories of how to analyze your own game and your opponent's. The chapter in which he analyzes four of Jimmy Connors' most important matches is a classic—you are hearing what the coach told his great player during the match. All players will find it exciting to be "in the huddle," listening to strategy and tactics discussed by one of the real masters.

### Play Better Tennis with Billie Jean King
By Billie Jean King and Reginald Brace. Mayflower, New York, N.Y. 1981.

As the preface states, this book is for players who do not need to be introduced to the rudiments of tennis, but who want to improve their standard of performance. It's filled with great photos and shows Billie Jean at her athletic best. The highlights are the informative and clear diagrams of court positioning for both singles and doubles. Billie Jean's love of the game is evident in every chapter, but the chapter "What Tennis Means to Me" is a delightful insight into her motivations and feelings about tennis.

### Stretching
By Bob Anderson. Illus. by Jean Anderson. Shelter Publications, Inc., Bolinas, CA. 1980.

This is an essential book. Not just for tennis players and not just for athletes, but for anyone who *moves*. Bob Anderson's approach differs from what many of us learned about stretching in high school: the bouncing, painful stretch. Bob teaches the static stretch, where you hold a comfortable position, then slowly extend it. There should never be any pain, and you shouldn't try for extreme flexibility. Every person is different, and every day is different. There are thorough instructions for hundreds of stretching positions, routines for different sports (including tennis), stretches to do every day to keep flexible, stretches to do while watching TV and stretches for the lower back. The book has recently become popular with orthopedic surgeons, chiropractors and sports medicine doctors.

### The Sweet Spot in Time
By John Jerome. Avon Books, New York, N.Y. 1980.

An exciting review of the latest efforts by athletes, coaches and trainers to maximize the "sweet spots"—those rare times when the mind and body are synchronized in perfect athletic performance. Jerome is a writer caught up in the excitement of his fitness age and has done his homework on improved physical performance and the latest scientific findings. He covers new concepts in weight training, nutrition, water needs of athletes, carbohydrate loading, and analyzes and explains recent scientific theories of movement, muscles, nerves, vision and motor skills. He concludes that improvement—in anyone—is possible and that with recent accrual of information and general understanding "... the stage is set for a massive revision upward in the limits of performance ...."

### Tennis for Thinking Players
By Chet Murphy. Leisure Press, West Point, N.Y. 1982.

Gallwey fans take note: Chet Murphy doesn't go along with the Inner Game concepts of letting your body go and doing entirely "... what comes naturally." There *is* thought involved says Chet. He uses his years of experience teaching and coaching to help you discover those thoughts that will lead to mechanical soundness. The book combines vivid word pictures (cues) with mechanical principles. There are many examples of how concentration and analysis have helped players get back into matches when they were playing poorly; they didn't turn off their minds but realized that winning tennis takes a combinations of "brains and brawn." This book will help all players come up with reasons why they're missing their shots and should help them make adjustments to stop the errors.

### Use Your Head in Tennis
By Bob Harman with Keith Monroe. Kennikat Press, Port Washington, N.Y. 1950.

Although there's a statement on the cover that this is "the ideal book for the weekend player," this book is valuable for everyone—from beginners to tournament players. It's full of great word pictures that help translate sometimes confusing concepts into more simple actions. The strategy and tactics chapters are lively and realistic—especially the sections on doubles and mixed doubles. Harman has great sympathy and understanding for the problems of weekend players, and for anyone who has been "overmatched" or "off-form"—in other words, everyone.

### Vic Braden's Tennis for the Future
By Vic Braden with Bill Bruns. Little, Brown and Co., Boston, Mass. 1977.

Vic Braden, the psychologist turned pro, has had great success—beginning with his teaching of young children at the Jack Kramer Club in Southern California—to his scientific research with Dr. Gideon Ariel. Braden has strong opinions about how the ball should be hit and backs up these opinions with lots of data and research. His book is a real thesis on the mechanics of hitting the ball and has enough of the Braden personality to keep it from getting too complicated. The serious student and player of the game will enjoy this book. Braden leaves very little to chance or your imagination. □

# *Index*

# Credits

### Editors
Lloyd Kahn
Charlotte Leon Mayerson

### Art Director and Book Design
Drake Jordan

### Assistant Art Director
Susan Sanders

### Photography (for Drawings)
Jack Fulton
Lloyd Kahn, Jr.

### Assistant Illustrator
Steve Rutherford

### Typesetting
Trudy Renggli

### Paste-up
Helen Jordan
Laura Riley

### Models for Illustrations
Beth Billings   Mary Rogers
Hugh Hansen   Sarah Stearns
Willa Denton   Bill Wright
Raphael Moon

### Photo Printing
General Graphic Services
San Francisco, Calif.

### Special Effects Photography
Chuck Rose

### Photostats
Marinstat
Mill Valley, Calif.

### Headlines
Type By Design
Fairfax, Calif.

### Proofreading
Susan Friedland

### Acknowledgements

*Thanks to the following who, in one way or another, helped make this book possible:*

Bob & Jean Anderson
Lesley Creed
Dave Garton
Charles Hoeveler
Leo LaBorde
Dave Maggard
John Marshall
Jeff Morse
Chet Murphy
Bob Richards
Jim Schwering
Rod Slifer
Dave Snyder
Bitsy Wright
Hilda Wright

# MORE WORLD-CLASS FITNESS BOOKS
# FROM SHELTER PUBLICATIONS

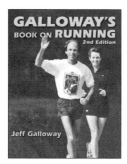

## Galloway's Book on Running
## 2ⁿᵈ Edition
### by Jeff Galloway

A complete revision of Jeff's classic book on running.

- 430,000 copies of original edition sold
- Training programs for 5K, 10K, and half marathons
- The second running boom
- New info on diet, "slow" running, clothing, and shoes

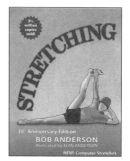

## Stretching
## 30ᵗʰ Anniversary Revised Edition
### by Bob Anderson

One of the world's most popular fitness books, now revised.

- 3½ million copies sold, in 23 languages
- Stretching routines for all sports (including running and everyday activities)
- 10 new stretching routines for office workers and computer operators

"A must-read for anyone who wants to stay supple for life."

*–The Washington Post*

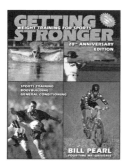

## Getting Stronger
## 20ᵗʰ Anniversary Edition
### by Bill Pearl

A revised edition of the best-seller on weight training. Of special interest to runners are off-season and in-season weight training programs for distance running and new rehab exercises for knees.

- 550,000 copies sold
- 80 one-page training programs
- General conditioning, sports training, and bodybuilding

"A must for anyone serious about fitness."

*–Newsday*

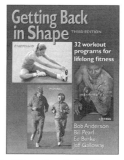

## Getting Back in Shape:
## 32 Workout Programs for Lifelong Fitness
### by Bob Anderson, Bill Pearl,
### Ed Burke, and Jeff Galloway

A unique workout book for anyone who wants to get back in shape.

- Stretching, weightlifting, and cardiovascular training
- 3-point programs

". . . simple programs designed for the busy schedule."

*–Kiplinger's Personal Finance* magazine